Management of
Bloodborne
Infections in Sport

Terry A. Zeigler, MA

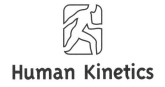

Human Kinetics

y of Congress Cataloging-in-Publication Data

Management of bloodborne infections in sport / Terry A. Zeigler.
    p.   cm.
Includes bibliographical references.
ISBN 0-88011-682-X
1. Bloodborne infections--Prevention.   2. Sports medicine.
3. Sports--Safety measures.   I. Title.
RA642.B56Z45   1996
614.4'4--dc20   96-44257
                                   CIP

ISBN: 0-88011-682-X

The publisher wishes to extend thanks to the University of Illinois for their cooperation and access during this project.

Copyeditor: Joyce Sexton
Proofreader: Erin Cler
Graphic Designer: Judy Henderson
Graphic Artist: Francine Hamerski
Photo Editor: Boyd LaFoon
Cover Designer: Jack Davis
Photographer (interior): Chris Brown
Printer: United Graphics

Printed in the United States of America   10 9 8 7 6 5 4 3 2 1

Human Kinetics
Web site: http://www.humankinetics.com/

United States: Human Kinetics, P.O. Box 5076, Champaign, IL 61825-5076
1-800-747-4457
e-mail: humank@hkusa.com

Canada: Human Kinetics, Box 24040, Windsor, ON N8Y 4Y9
1-800-465-7301 (in Canada only)
e-mail: humank@hkcanada.com

Europe: Human Kinetics, P.O. Box IW14, Leeds LS16 6TR, United Kingdom
(44) 1132 781708
e-mail: humank@hkeurope.com

Australia: Human Kinetics, 57A Price Avenue, Lower Mitcham, South Australia 5062
(08) 277 1555
e-mail: humank@hkaustralia.com

New Zealand: Human Kinetics, P.O. Box 105-231, Auckland 1
(09) 523 3462
e-mail: humank@hknewz.com

Contents

Preface

Because bleeding injuries are a common occurrence in athletic events of all types, it is important that people involved in athletics become familiar with bloodborne pathogens and know the procedures that can be performed to reduce the risk of transmittal. Recent research, however, shows that athletic personnel have been slow to respond to the threat of human immunodeficiency virus (HIV) and other bloodborne pathogens. A significant number of sports medicine personnel also are not adhering to precautionary measures that would protect them from the possible transmission of HIV and other bloodborne pathogens.

The key in athletics is to educate those working with athletes about the potential risk for HIV and hepatitis B virus transmission. *All athletic personnel* who come into contact with athletes must be responsible for themselves in their knowledge of Universal Precautions when dealing with injured athletes of all ages and with bloodborne pathogens.

The Occupational Safety and Health Administration (OSHA) guidelines were established to provide employers the information they need to make their work environment safe for employees who may come into contact with infectious materials. Some institutions have gone even further than the OSHA guidelines and have developed even stricter policies regarding the management of bloodborne infections. Employers should inform you of their own policies regarding bloodborne infections.

The purpose of this manual is to provide a foundational education regarding the transmission and treatment of bloodborne pathogens for all those who come into contact with athletes. This educational foundation will provide a basis and rationale for the Universal Precautions and procedures to be discussed throughout the manual. With the knowledge gained through this manual, all individuals working with athletes, young and old, will be better prepared to deal with blood in the athletic setting and to reduce the risk of transmission of bloodborne pathogens.

Acknowledgments

I would like to thank the following people involved throughout the process of writing this book, including Bob Wilson, John Bearden, and Joyce LaPointe. I'm also grateful for the help of Dr. Greg Landry of the University of Wisconsin and Dr. Malissa Martin of the Research and Educational Foundation at the NATA for their input as content consultants. I also wish to thank Linda Morford and Kent Reel at Human Kinetics for their work in preparing the text for publication. Above all, my thanks and gratitude go to my family who encouraged and supported me throughout the writing of this book.

—Terry Zeigler
Head Athletic Trainer
Southern California College

1

Bloodborne Pathogens

B loodborne pathogens are microorganisms present in human blood that cause disease in humans. These pathogens include, but are not limited to, human immunodeficiency virus (HIV) and hepatitis B virus (HBV). The prevalence of HIV and HBV infections has increased steadily over the past decade throughout the world. Human immunodeficiency virus and HBV infections can be fatal. Not only are these viruses capable of killing the host; they can also be transmitted through blood and body fluids to unsuspecting individuals. It is imperative that all individuals gain an understanding of the pathogenesis and transmission of these viruses so that the risk of spread of these infections can be reduced.

Hepatitis is a disorder involving inflammation of the liver. Common symptoms include loss of appetite, dark urine, fatigue, and sometimes fever. Hepatitis can be caused by infections and by toxins, including drugs; this discussion is limited to infectious causes. Progressive signs of infection are associated with severe fatigue, anorexia, nausea, vomiting, and jaundice. Fulminant hepatitis may result in hepatocellular destruction, encephalopathy, coma, and death (Buxton et al. 1994, 108).

Five different types of hepatitis virus have been identified. Hepatitis A virus is the most common cause of viral hepatitis. This virus is usually transmitted by food and water contaminated by human waste. It rarely causes serious complications. Hepatitis C virus (HCV) is mostly seen in people who have had a blood transfusion. However, with the introduction of blood screening, transfusion-associated HCV has been nearly eradicated in developed countries. Now the main route of transmission for HCV is parenteral (i.e., piercing mucous membranes or the skin barrier), and thus the precautions outlined in this book should be used to prevent transmission. Hepatitis delta virus, a peculiar virus that occurs only in association with hepatitis B, is common in the Mediterranean region. Hepatitis E is endemic in India and South America

("Hepatitis" 1996). Hepatitis B poses the most serious threat to athletic personnel, and along with HIV will be the focus of this book.

The risk of acquiring HBV infection is much greater than for HIV. Approximately 1,200 new cases per year are reported among health care workers, and 5% to 10% of those become chronic or fatal. Despite the fact that HBV is more contagious, public awareness is much greater for HIV. "Hepatitis B is as prevalent, if not more prevalent, and more infectious than AIDS," said Thelma King Thiel, president of the American Liver Foundation. "The public needs to know this" (Kong 1991, 1).

In 1992, HIV infected 40,000 Americans, bringing the number of HIV-infected people in the country to about one million, with a yearly death toll that exceeded 31,000. By comparison, each year more than 500,000 Americans become infected with some form of hepatitis virus, and approximately 16,000 die from complications of the virus each year (Stein 1993, 65).

Hepatitis B virus and HIV are transmitted in virtually the same ways, but with some distinct differences. While only approximately 8% of HIV infections in the United States are transmitted through heterosexual intercourse, 41% of HBV infections are spread through heterosexual intercourse. Although a majority of HIV infections can be traced to some type of risky behavior (i.e., intravenous drug use or unprotected sex), 26% of HBV cases have no known source.

Hepatitis B virus is more contagious than HIV because it is a hardier virus. Hepatitis B virus can remain infectious outside the body (for example, in dried blood) for a week or longer, whereas HIV is extremely fragile outside of the body.

Another underlying cause for the higher rate of transmission of HBV over HIV is that the virus tends to be more concentrated in the blood (100 times greater than for HIV). Because the concentration of HBV is so much greater, transmission may occur with smaller amounts of blood exposure (Stein 1993, 66). Hepatitis B virus can be transmitted through very small amounts of blood and through contact with saliva or other body fluids. Human immunodeficiency virus is not known to have been transmitted through body fluids other than blood.

Although HBV and HIV are not the only bloodborne pathogens, they pose the most serious risk to athletic personnel. The discussion that follows provides greater detail about HBV and HIV.

■ Hepatitis B

Hepatitis B virus is a contagious disease spread by blood products or by body fluids. It can culminate in liver failure, although only 5% of those infected suffer chronic liver damage ("Hepatitis" 1996). Type B infections have also been linked with a form of liver cancer called hepatocellular carcinoma, particularly in Asia and Africa (Sparks 1996).

Hepatitis B virus continues to be the single most important cause of viral hepatitis throughout the world. Hepatitis B virus is especially a problem when it infects a person together with HCV. Simultaneous infection with these two viruses is an important cause of chronic liver disease and hepatocellular carcinoma (liver cancer).

About one-half of the 300,000 people infected with HBV each year become acutely ill. The other 50% show no symptoms (or show minor symptoms similar to those of a cold) and usually never know that they are infected. The majority of newly infected people (90-94%) have immune systems that defeat the virus. However, 6% to 10% of adults (and 25-90% of infected children under five) cannot beat the virus and become chronic HBV carriers (Stein 1993, 66).

Chronic HBV carriers can transmit the virus to other individuals. Of chronic HBV carriers, approximately one-third will develop "chronic active hepatitis" which leads to cirrhosis, liver failure, and/or cancer. However, it should be noted that the chronic carrier can also be in an asymptomatic carrier state for years.

Transmission of Hepatitis B Virus

Hepatitis B virus has been isolated in a variety of bodily fluids including saliva, semen, vaginal secretions, cerebral spinal fluid, pleural fluid, breast milk, synovial fluid, gastric juice, urine, and feces. The most common mode of HBV transmission is percutaneous (through the skin) or via exposure to mucous membrane.

A large percentage (41%) of HBV infections are acquired through heterosexual intercourse. Transmission can also occur from mother to infant at birth, through the sharing of intravenous drug needles, and through blood transfusions. However, 26% of individuals infected with HBV have no known source of infection.

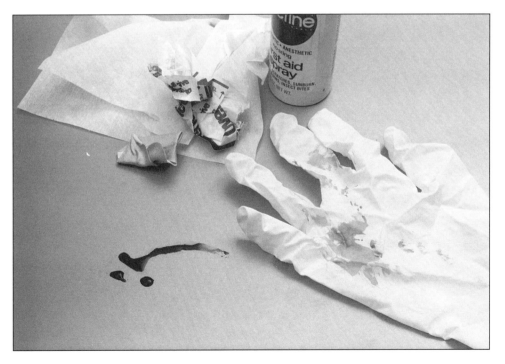

Hepatitis B virus can be transmitted through very small amounts of blood and can remain infectious for a week or longer, even in dried blood.

Hepatitis B Virus Prevention and Immunization

Prevention of the transmission of HBV can be achieved in the athletic setting by minimizing the risk of bloodborne pathogen exposure and adhering to Universal Precautions. It is of primary importance that all athletic training personnel (staff and students) be immunized for HBV.

The HBV vaccine was licensed in 1981 by the Federal Drug Administration. The vaccine is intended for preexposure prophylaxis. Two vaccines are currently licensed in the United States. The vaccines are administered in a three-dose series, with the first two doses given one month apart and the third dose given five months after the second. A postvaccination antibody test is available and should be given three to five weeks after the last vaccination to determine serologic response.

In late 1991, routine HBV vaccination of all infants was recommended in the United States. Internationally, more than 75 countries have included HBV vaccine in their immunization programs. Although only a small proportion of HBV infections occur among young children, they account for a substantial proportion of chronic infection and costs. Thus infant immunization appears to be an essential strategy for combating the virus (Francis 1995, 1242).

In 1991, the Occupational Safety and Health Administration issued regulations requiring employers to offer HBV vaccinations to employees with an occupational exposure to blood at no cost to the employees. Also in 1991 the Immunization Practices Advisory Committee strongly recommended immunization for all adults at increased risk of occupational exposure to HBV. Because of the occupational exposure to blood and bodily fluids in the athletic

Who Should Be Vaccinated for HBV?

The following is a list of individuals who are at risk for HBV and who would benefit from the HBV vaccine:

- All health care personnel having potential contact with infectious material
- Selected patients (i.e., individuals who receive blood transfusions) and their contacts
- Infants born to mothers with positive hepatitis B surface antigen or individuals who have had household or sexual contacts with chronic carriers
- Public safety personnel
- Users of illicit injectable drugs
- Prisoners
- Morticians
- Ethnic groups with high incidence of HBV infection (including Eskimos and Asian or Haitian refugees)
- Persons at risk due to sexual practices (i.e., sex with multiple partners, homosexual sex among males)
- Military personnel or travelers to locations where HBV is endemic, especially if staying more than six months

setting, all athletic training staff and students should be immunized before working with the athletes (Buxton et al. 1994, 108).

Some side effects may occur after an HBV vaccination and may last for one to two days. The most common side effect is soreness of the arm in which injection was given. Other infrequent side effects include flu-like symptoms with a fever over 100 degrees Fahrenheit, symptoms mimicking stomach flu that may be accompanied by abnormal liver tests, and sore throat or upper respiratory infection.

Hepatitis B Epidemiology

The World Health Organization listed hepatitis B as the ninth leading cause of death worldwide in 1994 (Perillo 1994, 34S). The threat of HBV infection is more widespread than for HIV. Hepatitis B is a disease of global distribution. It is estimated that there are approximately 300 million persistent carriers of HBV in the world, including more than 200 million in Asia (Umenai et al. 1994, 520). Of 35 countries in Eastern Asia and the South Pacific, 25 countries have an HBV carrier rate of more than 5%, with 17 of these countries having a carrier rate of more than 10%. In China, the carrier rate in the general population is 10%. In most of the island countries of the South Pacific, the HBV carrier rate is 10% to 20% or more.

Surveys suggest that there are more than one million HBV carriers in the United States (Perillo 1994, 34S). Cases per year in the United States along with deaths per year for all types of hepatitis and HIV are presented in table 1.1.

■ Table 1.1   Comparison of Cases per Year and Deaths per Year Between the Types of Hepatitis and HIV (Stein 1993, 68)

Type of hepatitis	Cases/Year	Deaths/Year
Hepatitis A	70,000	100
Hepatitis B	300,000	5,000
Hepatitis C	150,000	10,000
Hepatitis D	70,000	1,000
Hepatitis E	no test	0
HIV	40,000	31,000

■ Human Immunodeficiency Virus

Human immunodeficiency virus infects T lymphocytes in the human immune system. Because this cell is central to every phase of the immune response, its disruption cripples the immune system and leaves the body vulnerable to a variety of infections (Booher and Thibodeau 1994, 154; Calabrese and LaPerriere 1993, 7). Over time, the HIV-infected individual becomes increasingly susceptible to a variety of dangerous infections and malignancies. It is these secondary diseases that are the major cause of death for the HIV-infected individual (Calabrese and LaPerriere 1993, 7).

As seen under scanning electron microscopy, the HIV virus is shaped like a 20-sided soccer ball. The shell is made of protein, and the genes are contained inside the shell. Overlying the shell is a lipid membrane that is acquired by the virus after it infects the human host cell. Contained within the outer shell is another protein capsule. This cone-shaped capsule (the core) is made up of many protein molecules. All of the protective packaging protects the important and vital core: the genes and proteins that will help carry out the virus' reproductive mission.

The viral genes provide the instructions for making more viruses. However, the actual manufacturing of the genes and proteins needed to reproduce the virus is achieved by the chemicals found within the host cell. Like other viruses, HIV causes the host cell to devote its entire time to reproduction of the virus and renders it ineffective for its normal purpose and function (Hoffman 1994, 171). Human immunodeficiency virus is an RNA retrovirus because it has a dense cylindrical core that encases two molecules of viral RNA genetic material. It is a retrovirus because it possesses a special enzyme, called reverse transcriptase, that is able to make a DNA copy of the viral RNA. That enables the virus to reverse the normal flow of genetic information and to incorporate its viral genes into the genetic material of its host.

Human Immunodeficiency Virus Transmission

In order for HIV to be transmitted from one person to another, the uninfected individual must have an exposed portal of entry. The skin serves as a protective barrier for the body, so an open wound in the skin would create an entry portal for the virus. This wound could result either from an injury (such as a laceration) or through a needle-stick (purposeful, as in drug use, or accidental). The most common portals of entry for the virus are the vagina, anus, and blood vessels.

The virus thrives inside host cells. So one mode of infection involves passing an infected cell from one individual to another. Human immunodeficiency virus particles are also found circulating freely in body fluids of an infected

Who Should Be Tested for HIV?

The Presidential Commission on the HIV Epidemic recommended an HIV test for the following individuals (Rhode Island Department of Health 1989, 3):

- Any person who received blood or blood products between 1977 and 1985
- Any person using intravenous drugs, including people who used intravenous drugs since 1977 but no longer use them
- Any man who has sexual relations with other men
- Any person who has engaged in sex with more than one partner since 1977
- Anyone who has had sexual intercourse with a partner in any of the preceding categories, or with a person who is known to be HIV infected
- Pregnant women who may be at risk

The Three Stages of HIV

The course of this disease has been divided into three stages. The majority of people who are infected with HIV appear healthy and are unaware that they are infected (Seltzer 1993, 111). At stage I of the infection, the virus can be detected only by serological testing. Individuals with stage I infections carry the virus and can be infectious to others. Stage I can last from six months to 10 years or more (Calabrese and LaPerriere 1993, 7).

Stage II is referred to as AIDS-related complex or ARC. Symptoms may include (a) fatigue, (b) fever, (c) loss of appetite, (d) loss of weight, (e) diarrhea, (f) night sweats, and (g) swollen glands (Booher and Thibodeau 1994, 165). These symptoms may be persistent or intermittent. At this point, the individual is more prone to infection or malignancy. The level of HIV in the bloodstream rises and overwhelms the immune system.

Severe T-cell depletion in the presence of a major infection or malignancy marks the third and final stage of the disease. Most authorities believe that all patients who are infected with HIV will eventually develop AIDS and that HIV is ultimately 100% fatal (Seltzer 1993, 111).

individual, so another mode of transmission involves the exchange of body fluids from an infected person to an uninfected person, especially when the body fluid contains blood.

Although HIV is present in a variety of fluids, it is primarily transmitted through blood, semen, and vaginal secretions. Blood is the most concentrated source of HIV (Calabrese and LaPerriere 1993, 10). High concentrations of free virus are also found in cerebrospinal fluid and semen (Hoffman 1994, 172). Activities involving the exchange of these fluids between individuals also carry the potential for spreading HIV. Transmission occurs through the following methods: (a) sexual contact with an infected partner, (b) blood transfusion from an infected person, (c) sharing of contaminated intravenous needles, or (d) passage from mother to fetus through the placenta (Booher and Thibodeau 1994, 65). At least 97% of United States AIDS cases have been passed on through these four modes of transmission.

People who received blood transfusions or blood products between 1977 and 1985 (hemophiliacs and surgery patients) may have received HIV-infected blood. Most of the blood used for medical purposes during these years was safe, but people who received transfusions during the time have a low risk of acquiring the infection.

Transmission requires intimate contact between individuals. The virus cannot withstand exposure to air for very long because its membrane dries out quickly and deteriorates. For this reason, HIV cannot be passed along by the touching of a surface that has been touched by an infected person (Hoffman 1994, 175).

No scientific evidence supports transmission of HIV through ordinary nonsexual contact. Although HIV has been isolated in saliva, tears, sweat, urine, respiratory droplets, breast milk, cerebrospinal fluid, and amniotic fluid, there has been no evidence of transmission through these fluids (CASM 1993, 63; WHO 1992; Knight 1995).

There is also no evidence that HIV can be transmitted through swimming, pool water, communal bath water, toilets, food, drinking water, casual contact, mosquitoes, other insects, wrestling mats, taping tables, sinks or other surfaces, or through the air (CASM 1993, 63; NCAA 1991, 24).

There have been no documented cases of HIV transmission during athletic competition (Calabrese and LaPerriere 1993, 10; AAP 1991, 640; Mitten 1994, 63). In the athletic setting, only blood poses a degree of risk (AMSSM and AASM 1995, 510). However, athletes involved in anabolic steroid use could be at risk if they share needles (Seltzer 1993, 112). There have been two reports in athletes of HIV transmission secondary to injectable anabolic steroid use and sharing of needles (Sklarek et al. 1984).

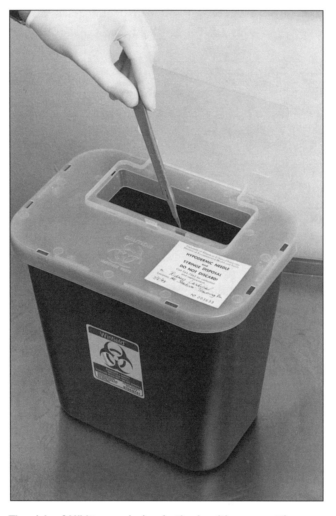

The risk of HIV transmission in the health care setting can be greatly reduced by careful handling of sharps. Dispose of contaminated blades, needles, and other sharp objects in a puncture-resistant sharps container.

The risk of infection is increased by having multiple sexual partners, by homosexual activities among males, and by sharing of needles among intravenous drug users. Heterosexual transmission in the United States accounts for about 8% of cases, but the percentage is rising. It is a significant mode of transmission in Africa and Asia. About 25% of AIDS cases occur in intravenous drug users exposed to HIV-infected blood through shared needles.

Transmission in the health care setting has occurred primarily through accidental HIV-infected needle-sticks of health care workers through hollow-bore needles. It has been documented that transmission of HIV occurs in approximately 1 of 300 needle-stick injuries involving infected blood (AMSSM and AASM 1995, 511). In a study of 2,042 percutaneous injuries involving HIV-infected blood, six health care workers were found to be infected. Of these six cases, five were related to injuries with sharp objects or needles. Only one was related to blood exposed in an open wound. All cases involved a large quantity of HIV-infected blood (Henderson et al. 1990).

Dr. David Rogers, a professor of medicine at Cornell who is vice chairman of the National Commission on AIDS, stated:

> In the health care cases, the infection in virtually every instance was caused by the transmission of large amounts of blood through hollow-bore needles. With cuts or scratches, the risk is as close to zero as possible. When two people bleed, they bleed out, not in. It's hard to imagine an exchange of enough blood to cause infection. (Kirshenbaum 1992, 13)

Human Immunodeficiency Virus Treatment and Prevention

Although a cure has not been found for HIV, new treatments are continually being researched and developed. The current primary treatment for HIV is a combination of drugs given sequentially to slow down the ability of the HIV virus to reproduce. However, further research needs to be done in the area of HIV physiology. Once the physiology of the virus is better understood, researchers will have a better understanding of how to design drugs to fight the virus.

Preventing HIV Infection

If an individual is currently not infected and abstains from sex and drug abuse, there is virtually no risk of acquiring HIV. If a person is sexually active, the risk of HIV infection can be reduced by following these guidelines (Rhode Island Department of Health 1989, 4):

- Use latex condoms for all types of sexual intercourse.
- Use a water-soluble lubricant with condoms to reduce the risk of tearing the condom. A lubricant also reduces injury to the membrane lining of genital areas.
- Use a spermicide containing Nonoxynol-9 together with a condom. This kind of spermicide kills the virus.
- Avoid anal sex.
- Do not have sex with prostitutes, with multiple partners, or with any partner who may be at risk for HIV infection.

Human Immunodeficiency Virus Epidemiology

It is estimated that one million people are infected with HIV in the United States (Davis 1992). This translates into 1 infection in every 250 Americans (AMSSM and AASM 1995, 510). Experts estimate that 1 in 100 adult males between the ages of 20 and 49 is seropositive (i.e., there is presence of antibodies [proteins to bind HIV] in the serum indicating exposure to HIV) (Seltzer 1993, 111).

Research indicates an overall seroprevalence of approximately 0.2% for the average college population (Hunt and Pujol 1994, 104). On the basis of this statistic, as many as 600 of the 320,000 athletes competing nationwide in varsity sports at four-year colleges could be infected with the virus (Bartimole 1995, 4). The age group of 20- to 29-year-olds is the fastest growing demographic group in the United States with a diagnosis of AIDS (Hunt and Pujol 1994, 102).

In the United States, 58% of AIDS cases are accounted for by homosexuals or bisexual males. Intravenous drug abusers represent 23% of United States AIDS patients. About 25% of all regular intravenous drug abusers are thought to be HIV seropositive (Seltzer 1993, 111). Only 6% of AIDS transmission is thought to be through heterosexual transmission in the United States; however, the World Health Organization reported that heterosexual transmission is responsible for almost 75% of AIDS cases worldwide (Seltzer 1993, 111).

■ References

American Academy of Pediatrics (AAP). 1991. HIV and sports in the athletic setting. *Physician and Sportsmedicine* 20 (5): 189-91.

American Medical Society for Sports Medicine (AMSSM), and American Academy of Sports Medicine (AASM). 1995. HIV and other bloodborne pathogens in sports. *American Journal of Sports Medicine* 23 (4): 510-14.

Bartimole, J. 1995. Preventing AIDS in collegiate athletics. *National Athletic Trainers Association News* (December): 4-7.

Booher, J., and Thibodeau, G. 1994. *Athletic injury assessment.* 3rd ed. St. Louis: Mosby.

Buxton, B., Daniell, J., Buxton Jr., B., Okasaki, E., and Ho, K. 1994. Prevention of Hepatitis B virus in athletic training. *Journal of Athletic Training* 29 (2): 107-12.

Calabrese, L., and LaPerriere, A. 1993. HIV infection: Exercise and athletics. *Sports Medicine* 15 (1): 6-13.

Canadian Academy of Sports Medicine (CASM). 1993. HIV as it relates to sport—position statement. *Clinical Journal of Sports Medicine* 3: 63-68.

Davis, K. 1992. Trainers slow to deal with AIDS. *Hartford Courrant,* 1 November.

Francis, D. 1995. The public's health unprotected: Reversing a decade of underutilization of Hepatitis B vaccine. *Journal of the American Medical Association* 274 (15): 1242-43.

Henderson, D., Fahey, B., Wily, M., et al. 1990. Risk for occupational transmission of human immunodeficiency virus type 1 (HIV-1) associated with clinical exposures. *Annals of Internal Medicine* (113): 740-46.

Hepatitis. 1996. *Hutchinson Encyclopedia* [online]. Helicon Publishing Limited: Oxford, Britain.

Hoffman, M. 1994. AIDS: Solving the molecular puzzle. *American Scientist* (March/April): 171-77.

Hunt, B., and Pujol, T. 1994. Athletic trainers as HIV/AIDS educators for athletes. *Journal of Athletic Training* 29 (2): 102-5.

Kirshenbaum, J. 1992. Uniformly uninformed. *Sports Illustrated* 77 (23): 13.

Knight, K. 1995. Guidelines for preventing bloodborne pathogen disease. *Journal of Athletic Training* 30 (3): 197.

Kong, D. 1991. United States to urge all children be vaccinated for hepatitis B. *Boston Globe,* 11 June.

Mitten, M. 1994. HIV-positive athletes: When medicine meets the law. *Physician and Sportsmedicine* 22 (10): 63-68.

National Collegiate Athletic Association (NCAA). 1991. AIDS and intercollegiate athletics. *NCAA Guideline 2H*: 24-25.

Perillo, R. 1994. The management of chronic Hepatitis B. *American Journal of Medicine* 96 (1A): 34S-38S.

Rhode Island Department of Health. 18 June 1989. *The way to fight AIDS: Nature of HIV infection.* Rhode Island: Department of Health.

Seltzer, D. 1993. Educating athletes on HIV disease and AIDS. *Physician and Sportsmedicine* 21 (1): 109-15.

Sparks, R. 1996. Hepatitis. *Academic American Encyclopedia* [online]. Grolier Electronic Publishing.

Sklarek, H., Mantovani, R., Erens, E., et al. 1984. AIDS in a bodybuilder using anabolic steroids. *New England Journal of Medicine* (311): 1701.

Stein, R. 1993. The ABC's of hepatitis. *American Health* 65-69.

Umenai, T., Takahashi, T., Goto, Y., Akiba, T., and Okabe, N. 1994. Prevention of Hepatitis B in Asia. In *Viral hepatitis and liver disease,* ed. K. Nishioka, H. Suzuki, S. Mishiro, and T. Oda, 520-21. Springer-Verlag: Tokyo.

World Health Organization (WHO). 1992. Consensus statement consultation on AIDS and sports. *Journal of the American Medical Association* 267 (10): 1312.

2

OSHA's Bloodborne Pathogen Standard

A committee of the federal Occupational Safety and Health Administration (OSHA) has recognized a need to provide regulations that would protect employees against health problems related to bloodborne pathogens. In December 1991, OSHA published a standard for occupational exposure to bloodborne pathogens in the Code of Federal Regulations as CFR Title 29, part 1910.1030; the standard became effective on 6 March 1992. This specific standard is considered to be a performance standard. This means that the desired results are stated and general guidelines are given for achieving specific results (Smith, Bott, and Holzrichter 1994, 1-4).

This standard requires all employers to take steps to minimize exposure of employees to bloodborne pathogens. To be in compliance with this standard, the employer must develop the following:

1. A written exposure control plan, to include
   a. the exposure determination record
   b. procedures for evaluating the circumstances surrounding an exposure incident
   c. communication of hazards to employees
   d. schedule for implementing methods of compliance
   e. postexposure follow-up
2. Implementation of procedures to control exposures
3. Initial training and annual retraining of employees with occupational exposure
4. A plan for offering HBV vaccinations and keeping medical records of the vaccinations

Step-by-step guides to developing an exposure control plan, such as *Bloodborne Pathogens Compliance Plan for the Educational Setting* published by Cramer, are available. These are excellent guides to follow in developing an exposure control plan for the athletic setting.

■ Who Is Covered by OSHA's Standard?

The OSHA standard applies to all employees who are exposed to blood or other potentially infectious materials through their workplace, including athletic settings. To determine who has occupational exposure, job classifications within the work environment must be reviewed. The exposure determination must be based on the definition of occupational exposure without regard to personal protective clothing and/or equipment. The Occupational Safety and Health Administration defines occupational exposure as such reasonably anticipated skin, eye mucous membrane, or parenteral contact with blood or other potentially infectious materials as may result from the performance of an employee's duties. This list is divided according to two groups of job classifications.

The first group includes job classifications in which all of the employees have occupational exposure. An example of an employee on this list would be an athletic trainer who is exposed to bloodborne pathogens on a daily basis as part of his job description. Specific work tasks do not need to be included for the workers on this list.

The second group includes those classifications in which some of the employees have occupational exposure. An example of someone on this list would be a coach. A coach might need to provide emergency first aid at times during the season, but it is not expected that this person would deal with bodily fluids as part of her job description. This list must include specific tasks and procedures that may cause occupational exposure.

A survey form can be given to all employees as part of a training session to help increase awareness of their contact with bloodborne pathogens. This form should contain the following information (Smith, Bott, and Holzrichter 1994, 7-3):

1. The employee's name and social security number

2. Job title and department

3. Job description

4. Tasks and how frequently they are performed

From this survey form, information can be collected to determine which categories the employees fall into. The first list should include all those employees who deal with occupational exposure on a daily basis as part of their job description. The second list should consist of all those employees who deal with occupational exposure on occasion and the tasks they perform that might involve exposure to bodily fluids.

Communicating Hazards to Employees

As part of the standard, all employees are to be trained and retrained by their employer. Training must occur at the time of initial assignment to tasks through which occupational exposure can occur and at least annually after that. If tasks are added or modified, additional training should be given.

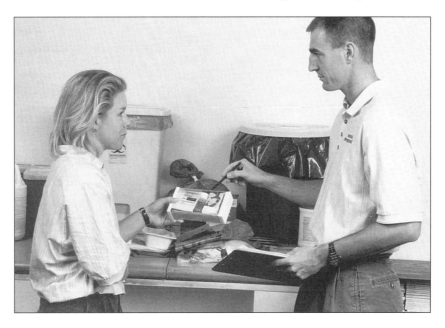

OSHA requires that employers train all exposed employees in the methods to prevent bloodborne pathogen transmission.

The training must be conducted at a level that makes it understandable to the audience and must include the following elements (OSHA 1992, 5):

1. Information on how to obtain a copy of the regulatory text and an explanation of its contents
2. Information on the epidemiology and symptoms of bloodborne diseases
3. Explanation of the modes of transmitting bloodborne pathogens
4. Explanation of the exposure control plan and how to obtain a copy
5. Information on how to recognize tasks that might result in occupational exposure
6. Explanation of the use and limitations of work practice and engineering controls and of personal protective equipment
7. Information on the types, selection, proper use, location, removal, handling, decontamination, and disposal of personal protective equipment
8. Information on HBV vaccination including benefits, risks, and availability
9. Information on how to report an exposure incident and on the postexposure evaluation and follow-up
10. Information on warning labels, signs, and bagging procedures associated with prevention and control of bloodborne pathogens
11. Question-and-answer session on any aspect of the training

▨ Keeping Records

A record should be kept of the training dates, names and job titles of trainees, and names and qualifications of the instructor as well as the content of the training session. The standard requires that employers maintain and keep accurate training records for three years. The training records must be made available upon the request of the Director of the National Institute for Occupational Safety and Health and the Assistant Secretary of Labor for Occupational Safety and Health. Training records must also be available to employees or employee representatives upon request.

Medical Records

Accurate medical records should be kept by the employee for the duration of employment plus 30 years. The medical records are to be kept confidential and are not to be disclosed to any person without the written consent of the employee.

The medical record should contain the following information on each employee (Smith, Bott, and Holzrichter 1994, 7-3; OSHA 1992, 16):

1. The employee's name and social security number
2. The employee's HBV vaccination status, including dates and any medical record related to the employee's ability to receive vaccinations
3. The results of all examinations, medical testing, postexposure evaluation, and follow-up procedures
4. A copy of the health care professional's written opinion
5. A copy of specific information provided to the health care professional

The medical records must be made available upon the request of the Director of the National Institute for Occupational Safety and Health and the Assistant Secretary of Labor for Occupational Safety and Health. All medical records must be kept in a confidential manner and maintained for the duration of employment plus 30 years.

Hepatitis B Vaccination Records

All employees who are exposed to bloodborne pathogens as part of their job must be offered an HBV vaccination, and a medical record of the vaccination must be kept for the duration of employment plus 30 years. If the employee refuses to take the vaccination, an HBV vaccine declination form must be signed by the employee and dated. This must also be kept as a permanent record. Figure 2.1 shows a sample HBV declination form.

Refusal of Offer of Hepatitis B Vaccine

1. I acknowledge that I am an employee of _____ considered to have a reasonable potential for exposure to hepatitis B and that the hepatitis B vaccine has been offered to me at no charge.

2. I decline the hepatitis B vaccination at this time. I understand that by declining this vaccine, I continue to be at risk of acquiring hepatitis B, a serious disease. If in the future I continue to have occupational exposure to blood or other potentially infectious materials and I want to be vaccinated with hepatitis B vaccine, I can receive the vaccination series at no charge to me.

_____

Name   Please Print

_____

Signature

_____

Social Security Number

_____

Job Title

_____

Date

_____

Witness   Date

■ Figure 2.1   Sample HBV declination form.

Exposure Control Methods Records

Documentation of methods to control exposures to bloodborne pathogens should be detailed in a written report. This report should include the biohazard tasks being performed, the locations where they are performed, procedures used to implement the control methods required (i.e., personal protective equipment used), and a cleaning schedule for the facility.

■ References

Occupational Safety and Health Administration (OSHA). 1992. *Occupational exposure to bloodborne pathogens.* Washington, D.C.: United States Government Printing Office.

Smith, T., Bott, L., and Holzrichter, J. 1994. *Bloodborne pathogens compliance plan for the educational setting.* Gardner, KS: Cramer Products, Inc.

3

Exposure Risks in the Athletic Setting

B ecause bleeding injuries can happen during athletic competition, there is a concern regarding the possible transmission of HIV and other blood-borne pathogens in this situation (Brown et al. 1995, 271). Any open wound can be susceptible to contamination with pathogenic organisms. A bleeding HIV-positive athlete could possibly transmit the virus to other athletes as well as to officials, coaches, and other support staff (Whitehill and Wright 1994, 114).

■ Risk of Human Immunodeficiency Virus Transmission

Although there has been no documented transmission of HIV during athletic competition, there is a theoretical risk of HIV infection from exposure to contaminated blood (AAP 1991, 640; Seltzer 1993, 109; Mitten 1994, 63).

There are no studies assessing the number of athletes who may be infected with HIV (Hamel 1992, 140; Davis 1992). However, as the number of infected athletes increases, the risk of transmission during athletic competition will increase (Leach 1993).

■ Risk of Hepatitis B Virus Transmission

There have been two published episodes of HBV transmission during performance of sports (Landry 1995). One involved five athletes in a sumo wrestling club in Japan; these members were exposed to an HBV carrier who had

The NFL's HIV Risk Formula

A study was conducted by the National Football League (NFL) to design a formula to determine the risk of HIV transmission during NFL competition. Information was collected from 11 NFL teams over 155 season games. Of the 575 observed bleeding injuries, 87.5% were abrasions and 12.5% were lacerations. The frequency of the bleeding injuries increased in association with games played on artificial surfaces and with a losing season record. The probability of HIV transmission was calculated as follows (Brown et al. 1995, 272):

1. 1 infected player per 200 players $\times$
2. 1 HIV transmission per 300 exposures $\times$
3. 0.41 lacerated players/game per 45 players/game $\times$
4. 3.46 bleeding players/game $\times$
5. 3.46 bleeding players/game per 45 players/game = 1 HIV transmission per 85,647,821 game contacts

This study puts the risk of HIV transmission in the NFL during competition at 1 in 85 million contacts. It is the only study of its kind, and further research needs to be done to check the validity of the formula as well as to study other contact sports.

dermatitis. The episode was reported in 1982. The other incident involved 568 Swedish track-finders over an eight-year period. Track-finders are people who participate in orienteering activities. Although the athletes may have been infected when they were scratched by tree branches that had been contaminated by the infected blood of a preceding competitor, experts agree that there was probably more than one mode of transmission (Landry 1995). There have been no documented cases in the United States of HBV transmission as a result of participation in sport activities.

Sport Guidelines on HIV

The guidelines on protecting athletes from HIV transmission vary from one sport to another. Because of the nature of the various sports, athletes involved in contact sports would be at a higher risk for infection than athletes in noncontact sports. According to the United States Olympic Committee's report on HIV transmission in the athletic setting, athletes competing in tae kwon do, boxing, and wrestling would be at highest risk for acquiring HIV infection because of the increased number and types of bloody injuries sustained in these sports (Goldsmith 1992, 1313).

Wrestling

Of all the sports, wrestling has adopted some of the strictest guidelines related to HIV transmission. Wrestlers infected with HIV are not allowed to compete in sanctioned events, and medical attendants who are infected are banned from treating bleeding athletes. If bleeding occurs during an event, the action is immediately stopped and the wrestler is treated. Blood must be cleaned from the mats and uniforms with a bleach solution, and cleanup materials must be disposed of in a biohazard container (Almond 1996).

Boxing

Boxing is handling HIV rather differently. Instead of stopping matches to stop bleeding, the sport is addressing the issue through testing. Five states require prefight HIV tests for boxers: Nevada, Arizona, Washington, Oregon, and New York. California has recently introduced legislation that would add California to the list (Springer 1996). The International Boxing Federation also requires fighters to present evidence that they are not HIV infected before title bouts (Brubaker 1993).

No HIV/AIDS educational seminars are offered to boxers by any of the four organizations that sanction world title fights. However, the World Boxing Council has distributed AIDS pamphlets and posters to gyms in 134 countries (Brubaker 1993).

Jeffrey Lawrence, director of the AIDS laboratory at New York Hospital, states that "there is much greater reason to test in boxing than in other sports. It's the only sport where there may be significant bleeding by both sides. That's not usually the case in basketball and football. In boxing, the wounds can happen dramatically and quickly" (Springer and Gustkey 1996, A3).

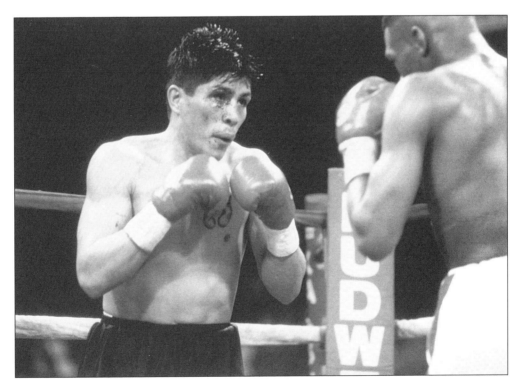

The risk of HIV and HBV transmission in boxing is greater than in other sports because there is often significant bleeding by both sides. Boxing is currently the only sport that requires mandatory HIV testing.

National Basketball Association

The National Basketball Association (NBA) has the most comprehensive HIV/AIDS program in sports. Annual seminars are funded by the players' association and are taught in each of the league's 27 cities by staff of the Johns Hopkins School of Public Health. These seminars are open to both the players and their spouses. A lecture is also given at the NBA's annual rookie orientation. All players receive an AIDS facts brochure and a five-tape video package entitled *Winning Against AIDS: The Official Game Plan.* Confidential counseling as well as HIV testing referrals over a toll-free hot line is also provided to the players (Brubaker 1993).

Serologic testing for HIV is voluntary and is encouraged in the NBA. Universal Precautions must be followed by athletic trainers and physicians while they are treating a player's wounds; and if a player is bleeding, play is stopped so that the athlete may be removed from the game for first aid procedures.

National Football League

The NFL provides all its players with a five-page HIV/AIDS fact sheet. The NFL also provides an opportunity for two players from each team to come to a league-sponsored seminar on drugs, steroids, and HIV/AIDS. These players are then expected to instruct their teammates on what they have learned. Testing for HIV is voluntary, and confidential counseling as well as HIV testing referrals is provided to the players through a toll-free number.

The only requirements the NFL has are that the athletic trainers and physicians wear gloves when treating bleeding players. The NFL has no policy dictating when a wounded player must leave a game or when he can return.

Major League Baseball

Major league baseball provides an HIV/AIDS seminar for all of the teams during one of their regular-season trips to New York. Rookies and minor league players are provided with separate seminars. Brochures on AIDS are provided for the athletes in both English and Spanish. Testing of players for HIV is voluntary and is encouraged. Counseling and HIV testing referrals are available to the athletes.

National Hockey League

The National Hockey League (NHL) has not developed an official HIV/AIDS educational program. Player representatives from each team were invited to attend a union-sponsored HIV/AIDS lecture in 1993. The league also has encouraged individual clubs to provide additional education for their players. The NHL had no HIV testing policy as of 1993. However, sports medicine personnel are required to wear gloves when treating open wounds on the players. Also, players are removed from the ice if they have a bleeding wound.

Figure Skating

Figure skating is the professional sport that has lost the highest number of athletes to AIDS. At least 40 top United States and Canadian male skaters and coaches have died from AIDS. Seminars are offered to the athletes at the United States Training Olympic Center in Colorado Springs. Testing for HIV is on a voluntary basis for these athletes.

National Collegiate Athletic Association

The National Collegiate Athletic Association (NCAA) instituted a bloodborne pathogen policy in 1988, which was updated in June 1994 (see appendix B). The policy stated that any player who is bleeding should be removed from the event as soon as possible. The player is not allowed to return until the bleeding has stopped or is under control. The NCAA does not restrict players from competing if they are HIV positive.

Although the NCAA permits HIV-positive players to compete, individual institutions have taken steps to reduce the risk of transmission in the athletic setting. In a 1992 survey that was sent to 860 institutions (with 548 responding), the following results were obtained:

- 33 (6%) had established policies on the participation of HIV-positive athletes;

- 15 others (3%) restricted participation in some way;

- 6 banned HIV-positive athletes from participating in any sport;

- 9 barred HIV-positive athletes only from selected sports such as ice hockey or wrestling.

There are no documented episodes of HIV transmission in the athletic setting. Boxing is the only sport that requires HIV serologic testing of participants and disqualifies those who test positive. No other sports or governing bodies require testing or disqualify HIV-positive athletes. Several organizations recommend temporary removal of the bleeding athlete from competition to reduce the risk of transmission of bloodborne pathogens. It should be kept in mind that the risks of acquiring a hepatitis viral infection from blood exposure far exceeds the risk of acquiring HIV in the athletic setting. Athletes are at a much higher risk of acquiring bloodborne infections outside the athletic setting than on the playing field.

■ References

Almond, E. 1996. Sports have varying guidelines on AIDS. *Los Angeles Times,* 31 January, p. C1.

American Academy of Pediatrics (AAP). 1991. HIV and sports in the athletic setting. *Physician and Sportsmedicine* 20 (5): 189-91.

Brown, L., Drotman, D., Chu, A., Brown, C., and Knowlan, D. 1995. Bleeding injuries in professional football: Estimating the risk for HIV transmission. *Annals of Internal Medicine* 122: 271-74.

Brubaker, B. 1993. In NBA, AIDS appears to faze few. *Washington Post,* 13 July, p. D1+.

Davis, K. 1992. Trainers slow to deal with AIDS. *Hartford Courrant,* 1 November, p. A1+.

Goldsmith, M. 1992. When sports and HIV share the bill, the smart money goes on common sense. *Journal of the American Medical Association* 267 (10): 1311-14.

Hamel, R. 1992. AIDS: Assessing the risk among athletes. *Physician and Sportsmedicine* 20 (2): 130-46.

Leach, R. 1993. The AIDS dilemma. *American Journal of Sportsmedicine* 21 (2): 169.

Mitten, M. 1994. HIV-positive athletes: When medicine meets the law. *Physician and Sportsmedicine* 22 (10): 63-68.

Seltzer, D. 1993. Educating athletes on HIV disease and AIDS. *Physician and Sportsmedicine* 21 (1): 109-15.

Springer, S. 1996. Morrison awaiting HIV test results. *Los Angeles Times,* 15 February, p. C1, C10.

Springer, S., and Gustkey, E. 1996. Boxer's HIV wouldn't have been detected in California. *Los Angeles Times,* 13 February, p. A3, A9.

Whitehill, W., and Wright, K. 1994. Delphi study: HIV/AIDS and the athletic population. *Journal of Athletic Training* 29 (2): 114-19.

4

Preventing Exposure in the Athletic Setting

S port personnel can help reduce the risk of transmission by following Universal Precautions and also through pre-event preparation. Universal Precautions is an approach to infection control in which all blood and certain body fluids are treated as if known to be infectious for HIV, HBV, and other bloodborne pathogens. These fluids include blood, semen, vaginal secretions, cerebrospinal fluid, synovial fluid, pleural fluid, any body fluid with visible blood, any unidentifiable body fluid, and saliva from dental procedures. Pre-event preparation includes providing proper care of existing wounds and making sure the necessary equipment and supplies are available to athletic personnel at the event, whether it be a practice or a competition.

By adhering to Universal Precautions and implementing the use of personal protective equipment, work practice controls, engineering controls, and housekeeping controls, sport personnel can help reduce the risk of transmission in the athletic setting.

■ Using Personal Protective Equipment

Personal protective equipment must be used if there are occupational exposure possibilities. The use of protective equipment helps prevent occupational exposure to infectious materials. Such equipment includes gloves, gowns, laboratory coats, face masks, and eye protection. In the athletic setting, gloves are the primary piece of protective equipment the medical staff will use.

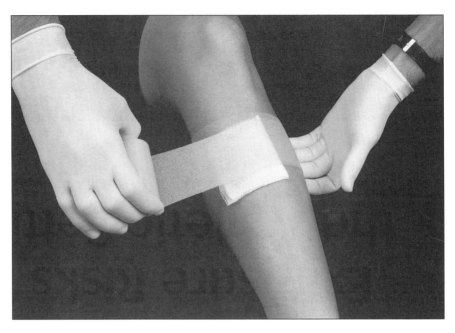

Covering existing wounds before competition reduces the risk of HIV or HBV transmission by blocking the existing portals of entry.

Universal Precautions and Pre-Event Preparation

Universal Precautions is the concept that *all* blood and certain body fluids are to be treated as if they are known to be infectious for HIV, HBV, and other bloodborne pathogens. This concept is fundamental to the practices outlined in the next two chapters, as all the procedures and tasks discussed are to be performed in a manner consistent with Universal Precautions.

Pre-event preparation is the first step in ensuring a safe athletic environment that reduces the risk of bloodborne infections. The route of transmission that athletics is subject to is mucocutaneous transmission. Although bleeding injuries cannot be prevented in athletics, the existing portals of entry can be covered to reduce the likelihood of transmission even when an injury occurs. The following pre-event procedures can be performed to reduce the likelihood of transmission from athlete to athletic trainer or from athletic trainer to athlete:

- All sport personnel should be educated in basic first aid and infection prevention and control (Arnheim 1995, 202).
- Medical and athletic personnel with existing wounds should cover the wounds with an occlusive dressing prior to the event.
- Medical personnel with exudative lesions or weeping dermatitis should refrain from direct patient care until the condition is resolved (CDC 1989, 20).
- Disposable gloves should always be available and should always be worn by a person who is working with bodily fluids (Booher and Thibodeau 1994, 151).
- Mouthpieces, resuscitation bags, or other ventilation devices should be available for use (CDC 1989, 20).

Latex gloves must be provided at no cost to employees or athletic personnel and must be available in various sizes. Hypoallergenic gloves and all other protective clothing must also be made available to employees who have an allergic sensitivity to latex gloves.

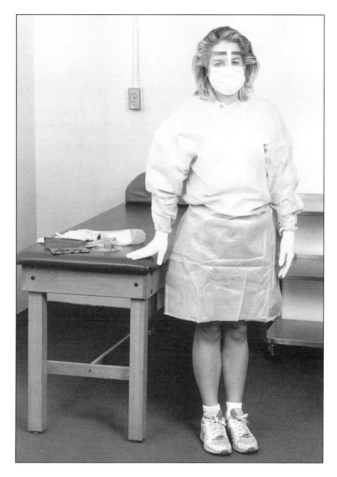

Proper personal protective equipment—such as gloves, gowns, face masks, and eye protection—helps prevent exposure to bloodborne pathogens.

■ Implementing Work Practice Controls

Work practice controls reduce the likelihood of exposure by altering the manner in which a task is performed. In work areas where a reasonable likelihood of occupational exposure exists, work practice controls include the following:

1. Restricting eating and drinking in potentially contaminated areas
2. Preventing the storage of food or beverages in refrigerators or other locations where blood or other potentially infectious materials are kept
3. Providing and requiring the use of hand-washing facilities
4. Washing hands when gloves are removed and as soon as possible after skin contact with blood or other potentially infectious materials has occurred
5. Removing personal protective equipment before leaving contaminated areas

Guidelines for Safe Handling of Protective Equipment

All employees should observe the following guidelines for safe handling of protective equipment:

- Remove protective equipment before leaving the work area and after a garment becomes contaminated.
- Place used protective equipment in appropriately designated areas or containers when it is being stored, washed, decontaminated, or discarded.
- Wear appropriate gloves when it can be reasonably anticipated that you may have contact with blood or other potentially infectious materials or when you are handling or touching contaminated items or surfaces.
- Replace gloves if they are torn, punctured, or contaminated or if their ability to function as a barrier is compromised.
- Never wash or decontaminate disposable gloves for reuse.
- Wear appropriate face and eye protection, such as a mask that has glasses with solid side shields or a chin-length face shield, when splashes, sprays, spatters, or droplets of blood or other potentially infectious materials pose a hazard to the eyes, nose, or mouth.
- Use respiratory assistance devices whenever resuscitation must be performed.

Procedure to Remove Contaminated Gloves

Contaminated disposable gloves should be removed in a systematic manner so that they do not contaminate the skin upon removal. To remove gloves properly, first use your dominant hand to grasp the glove on your nondominant hand at the palm (1). Then with your dominant hand, carefully remove the glove on the nondominant hand by slowly pulling it off (2). When the glove is completely off, hold it in your dominant hand throughout the rest of the procedure (3). Now carefully work your nondominant hand under the palm side of the glove on your dominant hand (4). Once you have worked the fingers of your nondominant hand to the finger holes of the glove on the dominant hand, use the fingers of your nondominant hand to grasp the contaminated glove and carefully pull it off (5, 6). Do this slowly so that there is no splashing of bodily fluids onto the skin.

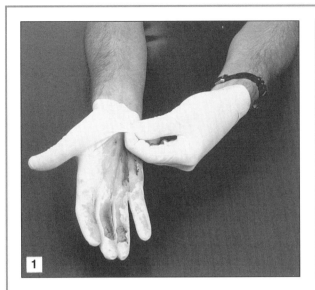

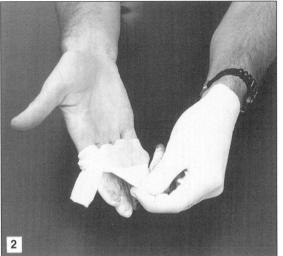

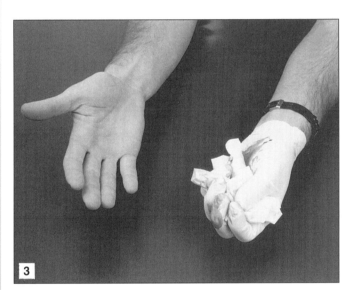

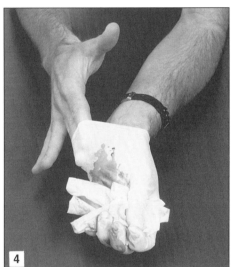

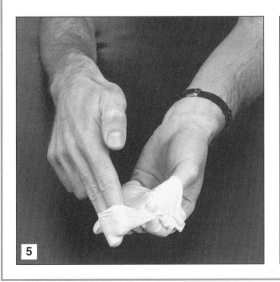

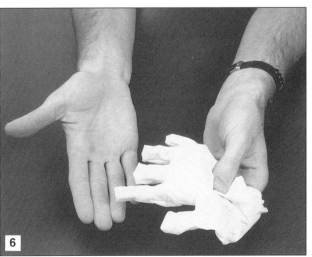

■ Implementing Engineering Controls

Engineering controls reduce employee exposure in the workplace either by removing or isolating the hazard or by isolating the worker from the exposure. Engineering controls include the following:

1. Sharps containers should be easily accessible to personnel and should be located as close as is feasible to the immediate area where sharps are used. Sharps containers must be puncture resistant, leakproof, labeled, kept upright throughout use, replaced routinely, closed when moved, and not allowed to overfill.

2. Reusable contaminated sharps disposal containers should never be manually opened, emptied, or cleaned.

3. Biohazard containers must be available and easily accessible to personnel. These containers must be marked "biohazardous waste" and be color coded. They should be constructed to be leakproof and closable.

■ General Housekeeping Practices

This Occupational Safety and Health Administration (OSHA) standard requires that the employer maintain the work site in a clean and sanitary condition. The employer must develop and implement a written schedule for cleaning and decontamination at the work site. This schedule must be based on the location within the facility, the types of surfaces to be cleaned, the types of contamination present, the tasks or procedures to be performed, and their location within the facility.

Several housekeeping requirements are listed in the OSHA standard. These include the following:

1. Clean and decontaminate all equipment and environmental and work surfaces that have been contaminated with blood or other potentially infectious materials.

2. Decontaminate work surfaces with an appropriate disinfectant, after completion of procedures, immediately when they are overtly contaminated, after any spill of blood or other potentially infectious materials, and at the end of the work shift.

3. Inspect and decontaminate, on a regular basis, reusable receptacles such as bins, pails, and cans that may be likely to become contaminated. When contamination is visible, clean and decontaminate receptacles immediately, or as soon as feasible.

4. Always use a mechanical means such as tongs, forceps, or a brush and a dustpan to pick up contaminated broken glassware; never pick up with hands even if gloves are being worn.

5. Store or process reusable sharps in such a way as to ensure safe handling.

6. Place all biohazardous waste in appropriately marked containers.

7. Handle contaminated laundry as little as possible and with a minimum of agitation.

8. Use appropriate personal protective equipment when handling contaminated laundry.

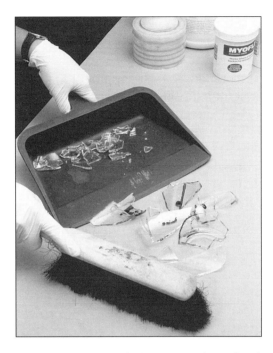

Always use a mechanical means, such as a brush and a dustpan, to pick up contaminated glassware. Never pick up sharp objects with your fingers, even if you are wearing gloves.

9. Place wet contaminated laundry in leakproof labeled or color-coded containers before transporting it.
10. Bag contaminated laundry at its location of use.
11. If clothing should become contaminated, remove it as quickly as possible and place it in the contaminated-laundry container for cleaning.

■ Labeling Containers Correctly

The standard requires that fluorescent orange or orange-red warning labels be attached to containers of regulated waste. The labels are not required when red bags or red containers are used, or if individual containers of blood or other potentially infectious materials are placed in a labeled container during storage, transport, shipment, or disposal In addition to being fluorescent orange or orange-red, the warning label must include the biohazard symbol and the word BIOHAZARD in a contrasting color.

■ References

Arnheim, D. 1995. *Essentials of athletic training.* 3rd ed. St. Louis: Mosby.
Booher, J., and Thibodeau, G. 1994. *Athletic injury assessment.* 3rd ed. St. Louis: Mosby.
Centers for Disease Control (CDC). 1989. Guidelines for prevention of transmission of human immunodeficiency virus and Hepatitis B virus to health-care and public-safety workers. *Morbidity and Mortality Weekly Report* 38 (S-6): 1-37.

Making Your Own Biohazard Kit

To make the containment and cleanup of biohazardous fluids easier, a biohazard kit can be easily assembled using medical supplies from the training room along with a leakproof container. The portable kit is designed to contain all equipment necessary for successful decontamination of an area. The kit is stored in the athletic training facility and is used on the benches along with the rest of the athletic training gear for home event coverage. The kit is also small enough that it can easily be taken from the training room onto the field or court for cleanup of an acute injury.

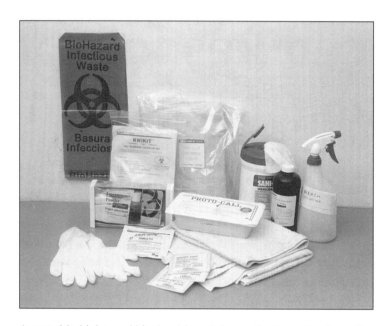

A portable biohazard kit should contain medical supplies from the training room. The supplies can be carried in a labeled, leakproof container to the field or court for cleanup of an acute injury.

The container needs to be leakproof and to include a lid. Large Tupperware-type containers can be used for this purpose. The container should be red; if it is not, it should be painted red for easy identification as a biohazard kit. The contents of the kit should include the following:

1. Disposable paper towels
2. Squirt bottle containing a 1:10 bleach-to-water solution
3. Hydrogen peroxide (to clean blood off of uniforms)
4. Small bag containing assorted sizes of disposable gloves
5. Small bag containing disposable gauze
6. Two small cloth towels (for containment of larger spills or wounds)
7. Red biohazard bag

5

Procedures to Protect Athletic Personnel

Athletic personnel need to know the specific procedures they can use to protect themselves from bloodborne pathogens. Whether handling contaminated laundry or cleaning floors and mats, athletic personnel should follow procedures that accord with Universal Precautions in order to protect themselves. This chapter provides specific instructions for dealing with contamination in the athletic setting. It also provides an injury scenario with step-by-step instructions that highlight the use of Universal Precautions.

■ Protective Procedures

Athletic personnel encounter many situations that put them at risk for the transmission of bloodborne pathogens. Sporting events often produce injuries, and these injuries are often attended by blood and other body fluids that may transmit bloodborne pathogens. By following the procedures that have been established by the Occupational Safety and Health Administration (OSHA), athletic personnel can minimize their risk of acquiring bloodborne pathogens.

Contaminated Instruments

Instruments that are contaminated with bodily fluids should be placed in a designated container for disinfecting immediately after use. Contaminated instruments should not be left on a counter where they could contaminate other instruments or materials. As soon as possible, the instruments should be disinfected with a disinfectant approved by the Environmental Protection Agency and cleaned in such a manner that manual contact is minimized. Disposable gloves should be worn throughout the process of cleaning the instruments.

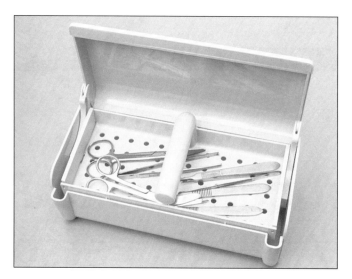

Instruments that are contaminated with bodily fluids should be placed in a disinfecting container immediately after use.

Contaminated Athletic Equipment

Equipment that is contaminated should be removed from the athlete and from the competition area as soon as possible. Depending on the equipment, a 1:10 bleach solution should be applied with disposable towels to clean the fluids off of the equipment. The equipment should then be wiped dry with a cloth towel before it is used again for competition.

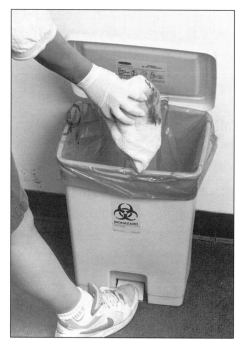

Contaminated laundry, towels, and equipment should be placed into a designated bioharzard laundry bag.

If the equipment is made of cloth (e.g., chest protector for baseball or softball), it should be placed into a biohazard laundry bag and laundered before being used again.

Contaminated Laundry

Most contaminated laundry in the athletic setting will be training room towels that have been used by athletes to wipe blood off of an injury. Contaminated laundry might also include uniforms, jerseys, and socks or any other part of an athlete's wardrobe. If the contaminated laundry is white, a 1:10 bleach solution should be prepared in a bucket to soak the laundry in before washing it in the machine. If the contaminated laundry is colored clothing, it should be soaked in a color-safe bleach.

To minimize the amount of contaminated laundry that will need to be washed, athletes should be encouraged to ask for gauze first to stop the bleeding of small wounds instead of using the game towels. Visiting athletes can also be encouraged in the same way through discussion with visiting coaches or athletic trainers about the use of gauze for small bleeding wounds. However, in the case of major injuries involving the need to control larger quantities of blood, applying pressure with an absorbent towel is a good way to contain the bleeding.

Biohazardous Waste

Biohazardous waste needs to be disposed of properly, and not through the regular trash pickups. Biohazardous waste should be collected by an established environmental control company. At a college or university it should be

What Is Biohazardous Waste?

Biohazardous waste is regulated and cannot be disposed of in ordinary trash bins. Examples of biohazardous waste include

- liquid or semiliquid blood or other potentially infectious materials,
- contaminated items that would release blood or other potentially infectious materials in a liquid or semiliquid state if compressed,
- items that are caked with dried blood,
- contaminated sharps, and
- other wastes containing blood or other potentially infectious materials.

Regulated waste does not, generally, include

- facial tissue or paper towels with spots of blood,
- adhesive or gauze bandages or wound dressings with spots of blood, or
- sanitary napkins or tampons.

picked up once a month and transported to the environmental control company's facility for incineration. A small monthly fee will be charged to the institution depending on the amount of biohazardous waste generated. Usually various plans are available depending on the size and quantity of waste produced.

There are also products on the market that allow biohazardous waste to be shipped through the mail in small quantities. These products are offered through various medical catalogs and represent a viable option if the amounts of biohazardous waste generated are small.

Sharps

Sharps include any disposable instrument (such as scalpel blades, needles) that have the ability to puncture the skin. Scalpel blades are used frequently in the athletic training setting and should be changed and disposed of after every use. Care should be taken during the removal of the blade so as to not cause any injury to the individual changing the blade. The blade should never be handled with the fingers. It should be handled with an instrument, such as forceps or a hemostat, and dropped into the sharps container. All used blades or needles should be placed into a sharps container for storage.

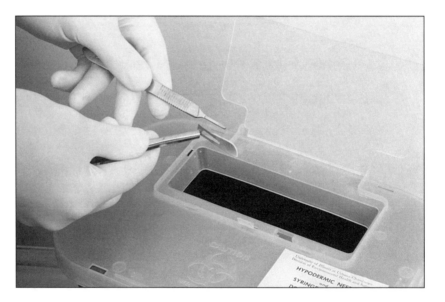

Scalpel blades should never be handled with the fingers. Use a forceps or a hemostat to remove the blade before dropping it into a sharps container.

Sharps containers should also be disposed of through a professional environmental control company. Disposal should occur and a new sharps container put into place when the existing sharps container is three-fourths full.

Contaminated Surfaces

Cleaning procedures for biohazardous waste should be performed only by individuals trained in waste removal. It is a common occurrence to have

How to Clean Contaminated Surfaces

Use the following procedures to clean up blood or fluids from contaminated floors, mats, or other surfaces:

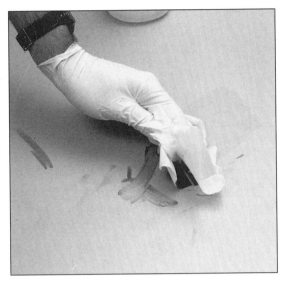

1. Use disposable paper towels to wipe the blood/fluids up off the surface. Place the towels in a biohazardous waste bag.

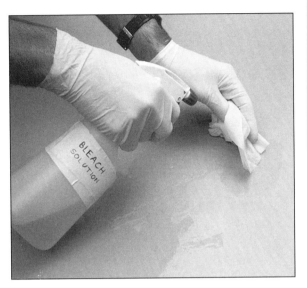

2. Spray the contaminated area with 1:10 bleach solution from a squirt bottle. Use liberal amounts of solution to ensure that the entire area has been disinfected. Place these towels in the biohazardous waste bag.

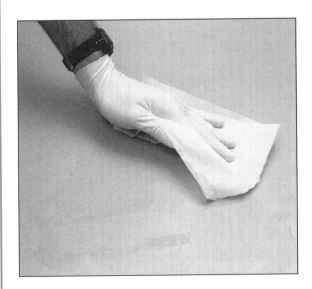

3. Use disposable paper towels to clean the area with the bleach solution. Allow the area to completely dry before competition continues. A dry cotton floor towel may be used at this point to speed up the drying process.

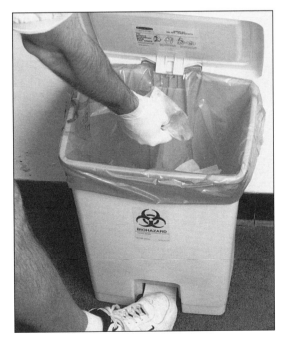

4. Place all contaminated materials in the biohazardous waste bag.

blood/fluids on the floor or other surfaces after an injured athlete has been taken care of. After the athlete is provided with the necessary first aid, the process of cleaning up the surface can begin. If the gloves worn to take care of the athlete have been bloodied, they should be disposed of in a biohazardous waste bag and a new pair of gloves should be put on. This will prevent the cleanup equipment from being contaminated when it is carried to the affected surface.

Bleeding Injuries

There is a risk that a bleeding athlete may infect another athlete. Follow these steps to prevent transmission of bloodborne pathogens from athlete to athlete:

- If a bleeding wound occurs during competition or practice, the individual should be pulled out of participation until the bleeding has been stopped and the wound securely covered (NATABOD 1995, 203; WHO 1992).
- Clothing or other pieces of equipment saturated with blood should be evaluated. Clothing and/or equipment must be changed before the athlete returns to competition (Arnheim 1995, 202).
- Occlusive dressings that would withstand the demands of competition should be used to bandage all wounds (Booher and Thibodeau 1994, 165).
- It is the responsibility of officials, athletes, coaches, and medical personnel to recognize and report a bleeding injury as soon as possible (Arnheim 1995, 202).

Postexposure Incident Procedure

The standard requires that the postexposure medical evaluation be made available immediately for employees who have had an exposure incident. An exposure incident is a specific eye, mouth, other mucous membrane, nonintact skin, or parenteral contact with blood or other potentially infectious materials that results from the performance of an employee's duties. Figure 5.1 shows a sample exposure report form. The person or persons who perform the evaluation and follow-up must do the following (OSHA 1992, 14):

1. Document the routes of exposure and the manner in which exposure occurred.
2. Identify and document the source individual, unless the employer can establish that identification is infeasible or prohibited by state or local law.
3. Obtain consent and test source individual's blood as soon as possible to determine HIV and HBV infectivity, and document the source's blood test results. If consent is not obtained, the employer must show that legally required consent could not be obtained.
4. If the source individual is known to be infected with either HIV or HBV, testing need not be repeated at this time to determine the known infectivity.

Universal Precautions Injury Scenario

In the following example, an injury scenario will be presented and the first aid steps to be taken by the athletic trainer will be outlined. The appropriate Universal Precautions are then cited in bold type.

Scenario—Two athletes collide on the basketball court while going for a loose ball. One athlete remains down on the court. This athlete is bleeding extensively from a two-inch laceration above the right eye.

1. On the way to the athlete, the athletic trainer surveys the scene and observes that the athlete is conscious and bleeding extensively from a laceration above the right eye.

The athletic trainer puts on a pair of sterile gloves while moving toward the athlete after observing a pool of blood on the gym floor and on the face of the athlete.

2. After the athletic trainer reaches the athlete, the athletic trainer applies sterile gauze to the eye and applies pressure to stop the bleeding. While applying compression to the eye, the athletic trainer proceeds with medical history questions and the appropriate questions to rule out concussion.

The athletic trainer then asks that the biohazard kit be brought to the floor by a student athletic trainer. When the student athletic trainer reaches the athlete, the student athletic trainer also puts on a pair of sterile gloves to assist the athletic trainer.

3. After the history is taken and concussion is ruled out, the athletic trainer moves the athlete off the court and over to the sideline to continue first aid procedures.

One athletic trainer stays on the floor to proceed with the cleanup.

   a. **The athletic trainer who is on the floor begins by cleaning up the blood off the floor with paper towels from the biohazard kit.**

   b. **After wiping up the bloody spill, the athletic trainer places the bloody paper towels into the biohazard bag that has been pulled from the biohazard kit.**

   c. **The athletic trainer on the floor then pulls out the spray bottle containing a 1:10 bleach solution and sprays it over the contaminated area of the floor.**

   d. **The floor is then scrubbed again with a towel to effectively kill any blood-borne pathogens that might still be on it. This towel is then placed into the biohazard bag.**

   e. **The floor is then wiped with a cloth towel to ensure that it is completely dry before play continues.**

4. After the appropriate first aid procedures have been performed on the athlete, the athletic trainer who has stayed with the athlete inspects the athlete's clothes carefully for blood. If the uniform is contaminated, the athlete is asked to change his uniform.

A biohazard bag is brought to the locker room to collect the contaminated uniform. The uniform is placed into the bag by the athletic trainer and then carried to and disposed of in the contaminated-laundry container.

5. Once all contaminated towels, gauze, etc. are disposed of properly, both athletic trainers carefully remove their contaminated gloves and place them into the biohazard bag.

After the gloves are removed, both athletic trainers thoroughly wash their hands with soap and water and then return to the bench. Lastly, the biohazard bag is placed into a biohazard container for safe storage.

5. Provide the exposed employee with the source individual's test results and with information about applicable disclosure laws and regulations concerning the source identity and infectious status.

6. After obtaining consent, collect exposed employee's blood as soon as feasible after the exposure incident and test blood for HBV and HIV serological status.

7. If the employee does not give consent for HIV serological testing during the collection of blood for baseline testing, preserve the baseline blood sample for at least 90 days. If during this time the exposed employee elects to have the baseline sample tested, testing shall be done as soon as is feasible.

8. Provide HBV and HIV serological testing, counseling, and safe and effective postexposure prophylaxis according to the current recommendations of the United States Public Health Service.

The employer must give the following materials to the health care professional who is responsible for the employee's HBV vaccination and postexposure evaluation and follow-up:

1. Copy of the OSHA standard
2. Description of job duties of the employee that are relevant to the exposure incident
3. Circumstances of exposure
4. Results of the source individual's blood tests
5. All relevant employee medical records, including vaccination status

▊ References

Arnheim, D. 1995. *Essentials of athletic training.* 3rd ed. St. Louis: Mosby.

Booher, J., and Thibodeau, G. 1994. *Athletic injury assessment.* 3rd ed. St. Louis: Mosby.

National Athletic Trainers Association Board of Directors (NATABOD). 1995. Bloodborne pathogens guidelines for athletic trainers. *Journal of Athletic Training* 30 (3): 203-4.

Occupational Safety and Health Administration (OSHA). 1992. *Occupational exposure to bloodborne pathogens.* Washington, D.C.: United States Government Printing Office.

World Health Organization (WHO). 1992. Consensus statement consultation on AIDS and sports. *Journal of the American Medical Association* 267 (10): 1312.

Report of Exposure to Human Blood or Other Potentially Infectious Materials

EXPOSED EMPLOYEE

1. Wash the exposed area thoroughly. Use soap for skin; use only water if eyes, nose, or mouth.

2. Notify your supervisor of this exposure.

3. Please complete this section. If you have any questions, please ask your supervisor.

Name: _____ Title: _____

Home Address: _____ Home Phone: _____

City: _____ State: ____ Zip: _____ Work Phone: _____

On _____ (date) at _____ AM/PM, at _____ (location),

I received an exposure to: [ ] blood [ ] other potentially infectious body fluid (specify, if possible:
_____)

This material came into contact with my:

 [ ] right/left/both eye(s)   [ ] nose   [ ] mouth   [ ] cut/scratched/damaged/punctured skin

This exposure occurred while I _____

_____

_____

I was wearing: **[ ] gloves   [ ] protective clothing   [ ] face protection   [ ] protective eyewear**

Immediately after I received the exposure, I:

 [ ] washed the exposed area thoroughly   [ ] reported the exposure to my supervisor

I **[ ] have   [ ] have not** been vaccinated against the hepatitis B virus.

I **[ ] can   [ ] cannot** identify the individual to whose blood or body fluid I was exposed:

Name: _____

Address: _____ Phone: _____

4. When you are finished , sign and date this section and give this report to your supervisor.

5. Promptly report to the health care professional to whom your supervisor refers you.

Signature of Exposed Employee _____ **Date** _____

cont.

Figure 5.1   Sample exposure report form.

EXPOSED EMPLOYEE _____   **EXPOSURE DATE** _____

SUPERVISOR

1. **Confirm that the exposed employee has washed the exposed area and has completed the form as completely as possible.**

2. **Complete the following information. If you have any questions, please ask your unit head.**

Your Name: _____   Title: _____   Phone: _____

On _____ (date) at _____ AM/PM, the above-named employee reported this exposure to me:

[ ] as described above

[ ] as follows: _____

_____

According to unit records, the exposed employee:

   [ ] has received [ ] 1 [ ] 2 [ ] 3 hepatitis B vaccinations **[ ] has not received** hepatitis B vaccination

   [ ]has [ ] has not received training in Occupational Exposure to Bloodborne Pathogens

Source individual identification **[ ] cannot [ ] can be confirmed**. _Complete a Source Individual Identification form._

I referred the exposed employee to the following health care professional:

   [ ] _____
         (list local health care professional here)

   [ ] _____
         (list local health care professional here)

Signature of Supervisor _____ **Date** _____

3. **Photocopy this form for your unit's records.**

4. **Send the original form and a copy of the employee's task description with the employee to the health care professional.**

■ Figure 5.1 _(continued)._

6

Education for Athletic Personnel

Prevention of the spread of HIV is closely tied not only to education about transmission of the disease, but also to education about and adherence to protective policies and procedures for sports medicine professionals interacting with the athletes. Athletic personnel can play an important role in reducing the transmission of HIV by educating other sports medicine professionals as well as athletes. In addition, athletic personnel can further reduce the risk of transmission of HIV by adhering to Universal Precautions when handling bodily fluids.

■ Educating Athletes

Bob Beeton, United States Olympic Committee senior manager for sports medicine, stated, "AIDS education at the amateur level is zero" (Hamel 1992, 141). It is important that education about HIV and prevention of HIV be emphasized to student athletes (NCAA 1991, 25). As Hunt and Pujol (1994) noted, "Uncertainty is often a precursor of unnecessary fear, and education is an important method for overcoming irrational fears while accurately appraising risk" (105).

An educational presentation should include information about (a) risk of transmission or infection during competition, (b) risk of transmission or infection in general, (c) availability of HIV testing and vaccination, and (d) the importance of immediate first aid for open wounds during competition (NATABOD 1995, 203).

Educational material can be included in films/videos, group instructional programs, pamphlets on responsible sex, pamphlets on HIV (myths vs. reality), posters, AIDS hot lines, professional counseling, and guest lectures (Whitehill and Wright 1994, 115).

Educational efforts can also be extended into the community to anyone who is directly or indirectly affected by the presence of bloodborne pathogens in relation to athletic competition (NATABOD 1995, 203). This information could impact all athletes in the community at all levels from recreational youth activities to highly organized adult competition.

The methods of instruction can be creative, but the message must be consistent and strong. Transmission of AIDS occurs primarily though unprotected sex with high-risk individuals and intravenous drug abusers. It is recommended that athletes be educated about abstinence, monogamy, the use of condoms, and other approaches to the prevention of sexually transmitted disease; about all the risks associated with nonmedical uses of injectable steroids and other drugs; and about the importance of not sharing needles, syringes, and other drug-related paraphernalia. The transmission of this disease can be reduced if individuals act responsibly.

Athletes who are HIV positive need to be provided with accurate information so that they are able to make informed decisions regarding their athletic careers. The decision to continue or discontinue competing should be made by the athlete, her physician, and a sports medicine professional (AMSSM and AASM 1995, 512). The variables that need to be considered include (a) the athlete's current state of health and status of HIV infection, (b) the nature and intensity of training, (c) the potential contribution of psychological and physical stress from competition, and (d) the potential risk of HIV to other athletes.

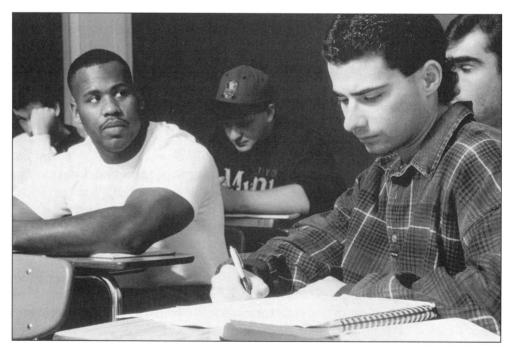

Education of athletic personnel is the most powerful weapon in the effort to prevent bloodborne pathogen transmission in sport.

◾ Educating Athletic Personnel

Several athletic organizations have emphasized the importance of education in combating the transmission of bloodborne infections in sport. The National Athletic Trainers Association (NATA) has published its own guidelines for athletic trainers. The American Medical Society for Sports Medicine (AMSSM) and the American Academy of Sports Medicine (AASM) have taken a joint position stand on bloodborne pathogens in sport that cites education as the most important weapon in the effort to prevent bloodborne pathogen transmission.

Educational Stance of the National Athletic Trainers Association

The NATA has published bloodborne pathogen guidelines for athletic trainers (see appendix C). In this document, the NATA is encouraging those athletic trainers who are responsible for developing educational programs to include information on various aspects of bloodborne pathogens.

An important ingredient for compliance is education. The NATA encourages appropriate education for student athletic trainers at all levels. According to the NATA, training and education of student athletic trainers at the secondary level should include the following (Bartimole 1995, 7):

1. Education and training in the use of Universal Precautions and first aid for wounds
2. Education regarding the risks of transmission or infection from the participants that the student athletic trainers care for
3. Education on the availability of HIV testing
4. Education on the availability of HBV vaccinations and testing
5. Education of parents or guardians regarding the students' risk of infection

In addition, training and education of student athletic trainers at the college or university level should include the following:

1. Education in basic and clinical science of bloodborne pathogens
2. Discussions regarding the ethical and social issues related to bloodborne pathogens
3. Information about the importance of prevention programs
4. Education concerning the signs and symptoms of HBV and HIV, as consistent with the scope of practice of the athletic profession and state and local law

Education will provide the foundation for a thorough understanding of why HIV is so devastating to the body and why it cannot be stopped at the present time. With this knowledge, athletic personnel will have a physiological rationale for the need to follow Universal Precautions to protect themselves and their athletes from the risk of HIV transmission.

The most difficult transition may be for athletic personnel who have been practicing in the field prior to the emergence of HIV. These individuals need to be knowledgeable about the risk of HIV transmission and learn to follow the Universal Precautions when dealing with bleeding athletes. This may require breaking some old habits. These people can do much to promote compliance with Universal Precautions just by following the precautions themselves. Athletic personnel who are established in the field can be positive role models for younger professionals. On the other hand, if experienced athletic personnel do not adhere to the precautions, younger athletic personnel may follow their example.

A combination of education and leading by example will be needed to improve the current poor compliance rate. It can be done, but the athletic personnel in the field will need to take a leading role and carry out the task.

Educational Stance of the American Medical Society for Sports Medicine and American Academy of Sports Medicine

The AMSSM and AASM feel that education of athletic personnel is the most powerful weapon in the effort to prevent bloodborne pathogen transmission in sport. First and most importantly, athletes should be educated on the risk of acquiring HIV and other bloodborne infections through sexual contact. In addition, they should be educated about the dangers of sharing contaminated needles and syringes such as those used to inject anabolic steroids and other drugs.

Education regarding the risk of transmission during athletic competition is also important. The AMSSM and AASM stress the importance of caregiver training in and adherence to Universal Precautions.

■ References

American Medical Society for Sports Medicine (AMSSM), and American Academy of Sports Medicine (AASM). 1995. HIV and other bloodborne pathogens in sports. *American Journal of Sports Medicine* 23 (4): 510-14.

Bartimole, J. 1995. Preventing AIDS in collegiate athletics. *National Athletic Trainers Association News* (December): 4-7.

Hamel, R. 1992. AIDS: Assessing the risk among athletes. *Physician and Sportsmedicine* 20 (2): 139-46.

Hunt, B., and Pujol, T. 1994. Athletic trainers as HIV/AIDS educators for athletes. *Journal of Athletic Training* 29 (2): 102-5.

National Athletic Trainers Association Board of Directors (NATABOD). 1995. Bloodborne pathogens guidelines for athletic trainers. *Journal of Athletic Training* 30 (3): 203-4.

National Collegiate Athletic Association (NCAA). 1991. AIDS and intercollegiate athletics. *NCAA Guideline 2H*: 24-25.

Whitehill, W., and Wright, K. 1994. Delphi study: HIV/AIDS and the athletic population. *Journal of Athletic Training* 29 (2): 114-19.

7

Ethics and Legal Issues

H uman immunodeficiency virus infection is a public health issue that has important legal ramifications. According to a 1991 report from the National Commission on AIDS, "AIDS is the most litigated disease in American history" (Perkin 1993, 45). Legislation has been focused on a variety of issues, including antidiscrimination, confidentiality, disease reporting, notification of disease status, blood center procedures, housing, insurance, education, counseling, prevention, quarantine, laboratory testing, organ transplantation, and labeling of bodies (cadavers).

There are three primary pieces of legislation that protect the rights of HIV-infected individuals. These are the Federal Rehabilitation Act of 1973, section 504; the American Disabilities Act of 1990; and the Ryan White Comprehensive AIDS Resources Emergency Act of 1990. This last piece of legislation helps provide outpatient funding and the financing of a health insurance program for states and metropolitan areas (Perkin 1993, 45).

Several controversial issues have come to the forefront in the search for ways to reduce the possibility of transmission of HIV in the athletic arena. These issues include mandatory testing of athletes, exclusion of HIV-positive athletes from competition, and breaching of patient confidentiality.

■ Mandatory Testing

Mandatory testing of individuals is currently being discussed and debated for a variety of subcultures, including health care professionals (physicians, nurses, dentists), pregnant women, premarital couples, and athletes. The Centers for Disease Control (CDC) had 8,871 reported cases of AIDS among health care workers or former health care workers as of 30 September 1992. That number included 243 dental workers, 903 physicians, 66 surgeons, and 1,937 nurses (Lyneis 1993).

The nation's largest medical and dental groups (American Medical Association and American Dental Association) oppose mandatory testing, as does the American Civil Liberties Union. Dr. Geraldine Morrow, past American Dental Association president, stated, "There is no scientific evidence to support the position that an HIV-infected health-care worker poses a real risk of transmission to a patient; there has been only one such case in the history of the epidemic" (Lyneis 1993).

A number of political, social, and professional organizations support mandatory testing of health care workers. These include the American Academy of Family Physicians; the American Federation of State, County and Municipal Employees; American Federation of Teachers; American Jewish Committee; American Nurses Association; National Council of Jewish Women; and the American Psychiatric Association.

The CDC officials believe that with the use of proper precautions the risk of passing the HIV virus to a patient in a health care setting is so slight that there is no need for a policy requiring mandatory testing. The CDC has also stated that health care workers with AIDS or HIV can continue to practice safely if they comply with voluntary restrictions on performing certain invasive procedures and also follow Universal Precautions (Lyneis 1993). According to a report from the New Mexico State Department of Health, the risk of transmission from a patient to a health professional is much greater than from a health professional to a patient (Lyneis 1993).

Courts have upheld mandatory testing of people who present a high risk of transmitting the virus, such as convicted prostitutes and persons who have possessed hypodermic needles illegally. Conversely, courts have invalidated mandatory HIV testing of people with a low risk of transmitting HIV or of individuals participating in activities that entail an insignificant chance of HIV transmission. Because the risk of HIV transmission during athletic com-

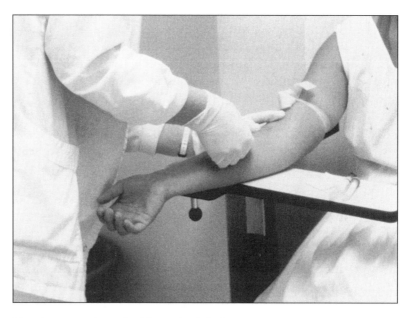

Mandatory testing of athletes for HIV is a hotly contested issue. Thus far, sports medicine groups have supported the policy of *not* performing mandatory testing of athletes.

petition is extremely low, mandatory HIV testing of athletes is probably illegal (Mitten 1994, 63).

The only sport that has mandatory HIV testing for athletes is boxing. Five states now require mandatory HIV testing prior to allowing a fighter to compete. Athletes who are seropositive are disqualified from boxing. Internationally, the World Boxing Organization banned a boxer from further competition after he tested positive for HIV before a fight in England in 1993.

To date, no athlete has challenged the legality of mandatory HIV testing. If it were challenged in the future, the courts would have to balance an athlete's right to privacy regarding his medical condition against justification for HIV testing (i.e., the low risk of transmission).

Thus far, sports medicine groups have supported the policy of not performing mandatory testing on athletes because the risk of HIV transmission in athletes is so small (CASM 1993; WHO 1992; AAP 1991; AMSSM and AASM 1995).

■ Exclusion of HIV-Positive Athletes

In 1987 the United States Supreme Court ruled that excluding a person with a contagious disease from an activity without supporting medical justification violated federal law (Mitten 1994, 63). The Americans with Disabilities Act of 1990 and the Rehabilitation Act of 1973 prohibit unjustified discrimination against people with HIV or any other disabling condition. These federal laws prohibit excluding an HIV-positive athlete from sports without a medically sound basis.

According to a brief filed by the American Medical Association, "the court held that exclusion from an activity must be based on objective medical evidence considering the nature, duration, and severity of the risk of infection of others, the likelihood of potential harm to others and self, and the chance that reasonable accommodation will reduce any risk (Mitten 1994, 63).

Reasonable accommodations that can reduce the risk of HIV transmission include the following:

1. Appropriate counseling
2. Warning all athletes of the possibility of exposure to HIV infection during any contact sport (without naming infected individual)
3. Removing bleeding athletes from competition
4. Following CDC's Universal Precautions regarding the handling of blood

The ruling does not justify categorical exclusion of HIV-positive athletes from all sports. However, the law does require a sport-specific assessment of the risk of HIV infection. Sports that have a higher potential for HIV transmission because of the high number of bleeding injuries would include boxing, wrestling, and tae kwon do (Mitten 1994, 63; Goldsmith 1992, 1311). Exclusion of an HIV-positive athlete from these sports may be legal with supporting medical justification, but this has not been tested in any court.

There is also concern about how exercise may affect the health of infected athletes. According to Landry, "The immunologic and psychologic benefits from exercise observed in healthy individuals with HIV infection appear to continue during the course of the disease, demonstrated by an increase in CD4 counts and CD4/CD8 ratios in the exercising individuals, and by a concomitant reduction in anxiety and depression" (1993, 1). A physician can bring about exclusion of an athlete if the athlete is medically unable to meet the physical demands of a sport. This could be the case for an athlete with a chronic illness for whom a physician is asked to assess whether sport participation would be harmful.

Because of the nature of HIV, asymptomatic HIV infection may not be a medically valid reason to exclude an athlete from sport participation. Mitten (1994) states that "current law is unclear whether increased health risks of participation to the infected players in a given sport justifies excluding them from competition" (64).

Athletic Personnel Infected With HIV/HBV

There is very little in the literature concerning HIV-positive or HBV-positive athletic personnel. The National Athletic Trainers Association has a section in its guidelines regarding the athletic trainer. According to the guidelines, infected athletic trainers may wish to

1. seek medical care and ongoing evaluation,
2. take reasonable steps to avoid potential and identifiable risks to their own health and the health of their patients, and
3. inform, as or when appropriate, relevant patients, administrators, or medical personnel.

Health Care Workers Infected With HIV/HBV

The medical community is also struggling over setting guidelines and restrictions on HIV-positive or HBV-positive health care workers. The CDC has decided to let individual states decide and assume responsibility for developing policy on HIV-infected health care workers instead of developing a list of exposure-prone procedures. In a letter of 18 June 1992 to state officials, the CDC reported that "exposure-prone invasive procedures were best determined by local review panels on a case-by-case basis taking into consideration the procedure, skill, technique, and if applicable, impairment of the infected health-care worker" (Albrecht 1992).

Each state has the task of coming up with its own guidelines regarding HIV-positive health care workers. The following, for example, are limitations placed on HIV-infected health care workers in Texas (Barton 1992, 52):

1. All health care workers shall adhere to Universal Precautions.
2. Health care workers with exudative lesions or weeping dermatitis shall refrain from all direct patient care and from handling patient care and equipment and devices used in performing invasive procedures until the condition resolves.
3. Health care workers who are HIV infected or HBV infected may not perform an "exposure-prone" invasive procedure without informing the

prospective patient of their seropositive status and obtaining the patient's consent beforehand, unless the patient is unable to consent.

4. HIV/HBV-positive health care workers may perform exposure-prone procedures only if they seek counsel from an expert review panel and have been advised under what circumstances, if any, they may continue to perform the exposure-prone procedure.

◼ Confidentiality

Physicians are prohibited by law from disclosing a patient's medical condition to third parties without patient consent or legal requirement. Third parties in the athletic setting would include coaches, athletic trainers, athletic directors, and officials. Legally, a physician could be held liable for unauthorized disclosure of an individual's HIV status (Mitten 1994, 64). The legal responsibility to warn the uninfected opponent would lie with the HIV-infected athlete and not the physician. It is also possible that the physician could be held liable if transmission occurs. This has not been tested in court.

The physician should be aware of state and federal statutes and regulations concerning confidentiality. Any physician who wants to know how to report a case or has related questions may contact city, county, or state health officials. Public health records are records maintained by a health department pursuant to specific reporting requirements. All states require that physicians report cases of AIDS to a health department; some require that cases of HIV infection be reported as part of their communicable disease reporting and control procedures. Some states also require that laboratory personnel report cases of HIV infection.

◼ References

Albrecht, L. 1992. CDC directs states to set policy on HIV-infected health-care workers. *Texas Medicine* 88 (9): 50.

American Academy of Pediatrics (AAP). 1991. HIV and sports in the athletic setting. *Physician and Sportsmedicine* 20 (5): 189-91.

American Medical Society for Sports Medicine (AMSSM), and American Academy of Sports Medicine (AASM). 1995. HIV and other bloodborne pathogens in sports. *American Journal of Sports Medicine* 23 (4): 510-14.

Barton, J. 1992. Laws address issues relating to HIV-positive doctors, health-care workers. *Texas Medicine* 88 (9): 52-56.

Canadian Academy of Sports Medicine (CASM). 1993. HIV as it relates to sport—position statement. *Clinical Journal of Sports Medicine* 3: 63-68.

Goldsmith, M. 1992. When sports and HIV share the bill, the smart money goes on common sense. *Journal of the American Medical Association* 267 (10): 1311-14.

Landry, G.L. 1993. HIV infection and athletes. *Sports Medicine Digest* 15 (4): 1-2.

Lyneis, D. 1993. The politics of AIDS: Health care, testing, secrecy, and AIDS. *Albuquerque Journal,* 31 January, p. A1.

Mitten, M. 1994. HIV-positive athletes: When medicine meets the law. *Physician and Sportsmedicine* 22 (10): 63-68.

Perkin, J. 1993. Facing the health-policy challenge of HIV infection. *National Forum: The PHI Kappa PHI Journal* 43 (3): 45-47.

World Health Organization (WHO). 1992. Consensus statement consultation on AIDS and sports. *Journal of the American Medical Association* 267 (10): 1312.

Definitions

AIDS (acquired immunodeficiency syndrome)—A condition of acquired immunological deficiency associated with infection of the cells of the immune system with the retrovirus human T-cell lymphotropic virus type III (HTLV-III).

AIDS-related complex—A collection of symptoms, including fever, weight loss, lymphadenopathy (abnormal enlargement of the lymph nodes), and the presence of antibodies to the retrovirus HTLV-III, that is sometimes associated with the later stages of AIDS.

antibodies—Any of the body's immunoglobulins that are produced in response to specific antigens and that counteract the effects of antigens especially by neutralizing toxins, combining bacteria or cells, and precipitating soluble antigens.

antigen—A protein or carbohydrate substance (such as a toxin or enzyme) capable of stimulating an immune response.

biohazard—Substance that carries a risk of transmitting an infectious disease.

bloodborne pathogens—Pathogenic microorganisms that are present in human blood and can cause disease in humans. These pathogens include, but are not limited to, hepatitis B virus (HBV) and human immunodeficiency virus (HIV).

contaminated—The presence or reasonably anticipated presence of blood or other potentially infectious materials on an item or surface.

dermatitis—An inflammation of the skin.

disinfectant—An agent or chemical that destroys vegetative forms of harmful microorganisms on inanimate objects.

engineering controls—Controls (e.g., sharps disposal containers, self-sheathing needles) that isolate or remove bloodborne pathogens from the workplace.

epidemiology—A branch of medical science that deals with the incidence, distribution, and control of disease in a population; the sum of the factors controlling the presence or absence of a disease or pathogen.

exposure incident—A specific contact (i.e., eye, mouth, other human membrane, nonintact skin, or parenteral contact) with blood or other potentially infectious materials that may result from the performance of an employee's duties.

hypoallergenic—Having a relatively low capacity to induce hypersensitivity.

immune—Condition of being able to resist a particular disease through preventing the development of a pathogenic microorganism or by counteracting the effects of its products.

occupational exposure—Reasonably anticipated skin, eye mucous membrane, or parenteral contact with blood or other potentially infectious materials that may result from the performance of employee's duties.

parenteral—Piercing mucous membranes or the skin barrier through such events as needle-sticks, human bites, cuts, and abrasions.

personal protective equipment—Specialized clothing or equipment worn by an employee for protection against a hazard. General work clothes (i.e., uniforms, pants, shirts, blouses) not intended to function as protection against a hazard are not considered to be personal protective equipment.

seroconversion—Development of evidence of antibody response to a disease or vaccine.

seropositive—Producing a positive reaction to serological tests.

sharps—Devices of any kind that can puncture, lacerate, or otherwise penetrate the skin. These devices include, but are not limited to, needles, intact or broken glass, intact or broken hard plastic, and intact or broken hard plastic devices containing blood or other potentially infectious materials.

Universal Precautions—An approach to infection control. Under this approach, all human blood and certain human body fluids are treated as if known to be infectious for HIV, HBV, and other bloodborne pathogens.

work practice controls—Controls that reduce the likelihood of exposure by altering the manner in which a task is performed (e.g., prohibiting recapping of needles by a two-handed technique).

B

NCAA Guideline 2H: Blood-Borne Pathogens and Intercollegiate Athletics

April 1988   Revised June 1994

Blood-borne pathogens are disease-causing micro-organisms that can be potentially transmitted through blood contact. The blood-borne pathogens of concern include (but are not limited to) the hepatitis B virus (HBV) and the human immunodeficiency virus (HIV). Infections with these (HBV, HIV) viruses have increased throughout the last decade among all portions of the general population. These diseases have potential for catastrophic health consequences. Knowledge and awareness of appropriate preventive strategies are essential for all members of society, including student-athletes.

The particular blood-borne pathogens HBV and HIV are transmitted through sexual contact (heterosexual and homosexual), direct contact with infected blood or blood components and perinatally from mother to baby. The emphasis for the student-athlete and the athletics health-care team should be placed predominately on education and concern about these traditional routes of transmission from behaviors off the athletics field. Experts have concurred that the risk of transmission on the athletics field is minimal.

Hepatitis B Virus (HBV)

HBV is a blood-borne pathogen that can cause infection of the liver. Many of those infected will have no symptoms or a mild flu-like illness. One-third will have severe hepatitis, which will cause the death of one percent of that group. Approximately 300,000 cases of acute HBV infection occur in the United States every year, mostly in adults.

Five to 10 percent of acutely infected adults become chronically infected with the virus (HBV carriers). Currently in the United States there are approximately one million chronic carriers. Chronic complications of HBV infection include cirrhosis of the liver and liver cancer.

Individuals at the greatest risk for becoming infected include those practicing risky behaviors of having unprotected sexual intercourse or sharing intravenous (IV) needles in any form. There is also evidence that household contacts with chronic HBV carriers can lead to infection without having had sexual intercourse or sharing of IV needles. These rare instances probably occur when the virus is transmitted through unrecognized-wound or mucous-membrane exposure.

The incidence of HBV in student-athletes is presumably low, but those participating in risky behavior off the athletics field have an increased likelihood of infection (just as in the case of HIV). An effective vaccine to prevent HBV is available and recommended for all college students by the American College Health Association. Numerous other groups have recognized the potential benefits of universal vaccination of the entire adolescent and young-adult population.

HIV (AIDS Virus)

The Acquired Immunodeficiency Syndrome (AIDS) is caused by the human immunodeficiency virus (HIV), which infects cells of the immune system and other tissues, such as the brain. Some of those infected with HIV will remain asymptomatic for many years. Others will more rapidly develop manifestations of HIV disease (i.e., AIDS). Some experts believe virtually all persons infected with HIV eventually will develop AIDS and that AIDS is uniformly fatal. In the United States there are 40,000-50,000 newly infected persons each year. There are 1.5 million infected persons in the United States. The risk of infection is increased by having unprotected sexual intercourse, as well as the sharing of IV needles in any form. Like HBV, there is evidence that suggests that HIV has been transmitted in household-contact settings without sexual contact or IV needle sharing among those household contacts.[5,6]

Comparison of HBV/HIV

Hepatitis B is a much more "sturdy/durable" virus than HIV and is much more concentrated in blood. HBV has a much more likely transmission with exposure to infected blood: par-

ticularly parental (needle-stick) exposure, but also exposure to open wounds and mucous membranes. There has been one well-documented case of transmission of HBV in the athletics setting, among sumo wrestlers in Japan. There are no validated cases of HIV transmission in the athletics setting. The risk of transmission for either HBV or HIV on the field is considered minimal; however, most experts agree that the specific epidemiologic and biologic characteristics of the HBV virus make it a realistic concern for transmission in sports with sustained close physical contact, such as wrestling. HBV is considered to have a potentially higher risk of transmission that HIV.

Testing of Student-Athletes

Routine mandatory testing of student-athletes for either HBV or HIV for participation purposes is not recommended. Individuals who desire voluntary testing based on personal reasons and risk factors, however, should be assisted in obtaining such services by appropriate campus or public-health officials.

Student-athletes who engage in high-risk behavior are encouraged to seek counseling and testing. Knowledge of one's HBV and HIV infection is helpful for a variety of reasons, including the availability of potentially effective therapy for asymptomatic patients, as well as modification of behavior, which can prevent transmission of the virus to others. Appropriate counseling regarding exercise and sports participation also can be accomplished.

Participation by the Student-Athlete with Hepatitis B (HBV) Infection

Individual's Health—In general, acute HBV should be viewed just as other viral infections. Decisions regarding ability to play are made according to clinical signs and symptoms, such as fatigue or fever. There is no evidence that intense, highly competitive training is a problem for the asymptomatic HBV carrier (acute or chronic) without evidence of organ impairment. Therefore, the simple presence of HBV infection does not mandate removal from play.

Disease Transmission—The student-athlete with either acute or chronic HBV infection presents very limited risk of disease transmission in most sports. However, the HBV carrier presents a more distinct transmission risk than the HIV carrier (see previous discussion of comparison of HBV to HIV) in sports with higher potential for blood exposure and sustained close body contact. Within the NCAA, wrestling is the sport that best fits this description.

The specific epidemiologic and biologic characteristics of hepatitis B virus form the basis for the following recommendation: If a student-athlete develops acute HBV illness, it is prudent to consider removal of the individual from combative, sustained close-contact sports (e.g., wrestling) until loss of infectivity is known. (The best marker for infectivity is the HBV antigen, which may persist up to 20 weeks in the acute stage). Student-athletes in such sports who develop chronic HBV infections (especially those who are e-antigen positive) should probably be removed from competition indefinitely, due to the small but realistic risk of transmitting HBV to other student-athletes.

Participation of the Student-Athlete with HIV

Individual's Health—In general, the decision to allow an HIV positive student-athlete to participate in intercollegiate athletics should be made on the basis of the individual's health status. If the student-athlete is asymptomatic and without evidence of deficiencies in immunologic function, then the presence of HIV infection in and of itself does not mandate removal from play.

The team physician must be knowledgeable in the issues surrounding the management of HIV-infected student-athletes. HIV must be recognized as a potentially chronic disease, frequently affording the affected individual many years of excellent health and productive life during its natural history. During this period of preserved health, the team physician may be involved in a series of complex issues surrounding the advisability of continued exercise and athletics competition.

The decision to advise continued athletics competition should involve the student-athlete, the student-athlete's personal physician and the team physician. Variables to be considered in reaching the decision include the student-athlete's current state of health and the status of his/her HIV infection, the nature and intensity of his/her training, and potential contribution of stress from athletics competition to deterioration of his/her health status.

There is no evidence that exercise and training of moderate intensity is harmful to the health of HIV-infected individuals. Unfortunately, there are no data looking at the effects of intense training and competition at an elite, highly competitive level on the HIV-infected student-athlete.

Disease Transmission—Concerns of transmission in athletics revolve around exposure to contaminated blood through open wounds or mucous membranes. Precise risk of such transmission is impossible to calculate but epidemiologic and biologic evidence suggests that it is extremely low (see section on comparison of HBV/HIV). There have been no validated reports of transmission of HIV in the athletics setting.[3,13] Therefore, there is no recommended restriction of student-athletes merely because they are infected with HIV.

Administrative Issues

The identity of individuals infected with a blood-borne pathogen must remain confidential. Only those persons in whom the infected student chooses to confide have a right to know about this aspect of the student's medical history. This confidentiality must be respected in every case and at all times by college officials, including coaches, unless the student chooses to make the fact public.

Athletics Health-Care Responsibilities

The following recommendations are designed to further minimize risk of blood-borne pathogen transmission in the context of athletics events and to provide treatment guidelines for care givers. These are sometimes referred to as "universal precautions," but some additions and modifications have been made as relevant to the athletics arena.

1. Pre-event preparation includes proper care for existing wounds, abrasions, cuts or weeping wounds that may serve as a source of bleeding or as a port of entry for blood-borne pathogens. These wounds should be covered with an occlusive dressing that will withstand the demands of competition. Likewise, care providers with healing wounds or dermatitis should have these areas adequately covered to prevent transmission to or from a participant. Student-athletes may be advised to wear more protective equipment on high-risk areas, such as elbows and hands.

2. The necessary equipment and/or supplies important for compliance with universal precautions should be available to care givers. These supplies include appropriate gloves, disinfectant bleach, antiseptics, designated receptacles for soiled equipment and uniforms, bandages and/or dressings and a container for appropriate disposal of needles, syringes or scalpels.

3. When a student-athlete is bleeding, the bleeding must be stopped and the open wound covered with a dressing sturdy enough to withstand the demands of activity before the student-athlete may continue participation in practice or competition. Current NCAA policy mandates the immediate, aggressive treatment of open wounds or skin lesions that are deemed potential risks for transmission of disease. Participants with active bleeding should be removed from the event as soon as is practical. Return to play is determined by appropriate medical staff personnel. Any participant whose uniform is saturated with blood, regardless of the source, must have that uniform evaluated by appropriate medical personnel for potential infectivity and changed if necessary before return to participation.

4. During an event, early recognition of uncontrolled bleeding is the responsibility of officials, student-athletes, coaches and medical personnel. In particular, student-athletes should be aware of their responsibility to report a bleeding wound to the proper medical personnel.

5. Personnel managing an acute blood exposure must follow the guidelines for universal precaution. Sterile latex gloves should be worn for direct contact with blood or body fluids containing blood. Gloves should be changed after treating each individual participant and after glove removal, hands should be washed.

6. Any surface contaminated with spilled blood should be cleaned in accordance with the following procedures: With gloves on, the spill should be contained in as small an area as possible. After the blood is removed, the surface area of concern should be cleaned with an appropriate decontaminate.

7. Proper disposal procedures should be practiced to prevent injuries caused by needles, scalpels and other sharp instruments or devices.

8. After each practice or game, any equipment or uniforms soiled with blood should be handled and laundered in accordance with hygienic methods normally used for treatment of any soiled equipment or clothing before subsequent use. This includes provisions for bagging the soiled items in a manner to prevent secondary contamination of other items or personnel.

9. Finally, all personnel involved with sports should be trained in basic first aid and infection control, including the preventive measures outlined previously.

Member institutions should ensure that policies exist for orientation and education of all health-care workers on the prevention and transmission of blood-borne pathogens. Additionally, in 1992, the Occupational Safety and Health Administration (OSHA) developed a standard directed to eliminating or minimizing occupational exposure to blood-borne pathogens. Many of the recommendations included in this guideline are part of the standard. Each member institution should determine the applicability of the OSHA standard to its personnel and facilities.

References

1. AIDS education on the college campus: A theme issue. *Journal of American College Health* 40(2):51-100. 1991.

2. American Academy of Pediatrics: Human immunodeficiency virus (AIDS virus) in the athletic setting. *Pediatrics* 88(3):640-641. 1991.

3. Calabrese L. et al.: HIV infections: exercise and athletes. *Sports Medicine* 15(1):1-7. 1993.

4. Canadian Academy of Sports Medicine position statement: HIV as it relates to sport. *Clinical Journal of Sports Medicine* 3:63-68. 1993.

5. Fitzgibbon J. et al.: Transmissions from one child to another of human immunodeficiency virus type I with a zidovudine-resistance mutation. *New England Journal of Medicine* 329(25):1835-1841. 1993.

6. HIV transmission between two adolescent brothers with hemophilia. *Morbidity and Mortality Weekly Report* 42(49):948-951. 1993.

7. Kashiwagi S. et al.: Outbreak of hepatitis B in members of a highschool sumo wrestling club. *Journal of American Medical Association* 248(2):213-214. 1982.

8. Klein R.S., Freidland G.H.: Transmission of human immunodeficiency virus type 1 (HIV-1) by exposure to blood: defining the risk. *Annals of Internal Medicine* 113(10):729-730. 1990.

9. Public health services guidelines for counseling and antibody testing to prevent HIV infection and AIDS. *Morbidity and Mortality Weekly Report* 36(31):509-515. 1987.

10. Recommendations for prevention of HIV transmission in health care settings. *Morbidity and Mortality Weekly Report* 36(25):3S-18S. 1987.

11. United States Olympic Committee Sports Medicine and Science Committee: Transmission of infectious agents during athletic competition. 1991. (1750 East Boulder Street, Colorado Springs, CO 80909).

12. Update: Universal precautions for prevention of transmission by human immunodeficiency virus, Hepatitis B virus, and other blood borne pathogens in health care settings. *Morbidity and Mortality Weekly Report* 37:377-388. 1988.

13. When sports and HIV share the bill, smart money goes on common sense. *Journal of American Medical Association* 267(10):1311-1314. 1992.

14. World Health Organization consensus statement: Consultation on AIDS and sports. *Journal of American Medical Association* 267(10): 1312. 1992.

15. The AOSSM and AMSSM position on HIV and other blood-borne pathogens in sports. 1993. (American Orthopaedic Society for Sports Medicine, 230 Calvary Street, Waltham, MA 02154).

NATA Bloodborne Pathogens Guidelines for Athletic Trainers

The NATA recognizes that blood borne pathogens such as HIV, HBV, and HCV present many complex issues for athletic trainers, athletic administrators, and others involved with the care and training of athletes. As the primary health care profession involved with the physically active, it is important for athletic trainers to be aware of these issues. The NATA therefore offers the following guidelines and information concerning the management of blood borne pathogen-related issues in the context of athletics and settings in which the physically active are involved.

It is essential to remember, however, that the medical, legal, and professional knowledge, standards, and requirements concerning blood borne pathogens are changing and evolving constantly, and vary, in addition, from place to place and from setting to setting. The guidance provided in these guidelines must not, therefore, be taken to represent national standards applicable to members of the NATA. Rather, the guidance here is intended to highlight issues, problems and potential approaches to (or management of) those problems that NATA members can consider when developing their own policies with respect to management of these issues.

Athletic Participation

Decisions regarding the participation of athletes infected with blood borne pathogens in athletic competitions should be made on an individual basis, following the standard or appropriate procedures generally followed with respect to health-related participation questions, and taking into account only those factors that are directly relevant to the health and rights of the athlete, the other participants in the competition, and the other constituencies with interests in the competition, the athletic program, the athletes, and the sponsoring schools or organizations.

The following are examples of factors that are appropriate in many settings to the decision-making process:

1. The current health of the athlete

2. The nature and intensity of the athlete's training

3. The physiological effects of the athletic competition

4. The potential risks of the infection being transmitted

5. The desires of the athlete

6. The administrative and legal needs of the competitive program

Education of the Physically Active

In a rapidly changing medical, social, and legal environment, educational information concerning blood borne pathogens is of particular importance. *The athletic trainer should play a role with respect to the creation and dissemination of educational information that is appropriate to and particularized with respect to that athletic trainer's position and responsibilities.*

Athletic trainers who are responsible for developing educational programs with respect to blood borne pathogens should provide appropriate information concerning:

1. The risk of transmission or infection during competition

2. The risk of transmission or infection generally

3. The availability of HIV testing

4. The availability of HBV testing and vaccinations

Athletic trainers who have educational program responsibility should extend educational efforts to include those, such as athletes' families and communities, who are directly or indirectly affected by the presence of blood borne pathogens in athletic competitions.

All education activities should, of course, be limited to those within athletic trainers' scope of practice and competence, be within their job descriptions or other relevant roles, and be undertaken with the cooperation and/or consent of appropriate personnel, such as team physicians, coaches, athletic directors, school or institutional counsel, and school and community leaders.

The Athletic Trainer and Blood Borne Pathogens at Athletic Events

The risk of blood borne pathogen transmission at athletic events is directly associated with contact with blood or other body fluids. Athletic trainers who have responsibility for overseeing events at which such contact is possible should use appropriate preventative measures and be prepared to administer appropriate treatment, consistent with the requirements and restrictions of their jobs, and local, state, and federal law.

In most cases, these measures will include:

1. Pre-event care and covering of existing wounds, cuts, and abrasions

2. Provision of the necessary or usual equipment and supplies for compliance with universal precautions, including, for example, latex gloves, biohazard containers, disinfectants, bleach solutions, antiseptics, and sharps containers

3. Early recognition and control of a bleeding athlete, including measures such as appropriate cleaning and covering procedures, or changing of blood-saturated clothes

4. Requiring all athletes to report all wounds immediately

5. Insistence that universal precaution guidelines be followed at all times in the management of acute blood exposure

6. Appropriate cleaning and disposal policies and procedures for contaminated areas or equipment

7. Appropriate policies with respect to the delivery of life-saving techniques in the absence of protective equipment

8. Post-event management including, as appropriate, re-evaluation, coverage of wounds, cuts, and abrasions

9. Appropriate policy development, including incorporation, with necessary legal and administrative assistance, of existing OSHA and other legal guidelines and conference or school rules and regulations

Student Athletic Trainer Education

NATA encourages appropriate education of and involvement of the student athletic trainer in educational efforts involving blood borne pathogens. These efforts and programs will vary significantly based on local needs, requirements, resources and policies.

At the secondary school level, educational efforts should include items such as the following:

1. Education and training in the use of universal precautions and first aid for wounds

2. Education regarding the risks of transmission/infection from the participants that they care for

3. Education on the availability of HIV testing

4. Education on the availability of HBV vaccinations and testing

5. Education of parents or guardians regarding the students' risk of infection

At the college or university level, education efforts should include items such as those listed above, and, additionally, as appropriate, the following:

1. Education in basic and clinical science of blood borne pathogens

2. Discussions regarding the ethical and social issues related to blood borne pathogens

3. The importance of prevention programs

4. Education concerning the signs and symptoms of HBV and HIV, as consistent with the scope of practice of the athletic profession and state and local law

Universal Precautions and OSHA Regulations

Athletic trainers should, consistent with their job descriptions and the time and legal requirements and limitations of their jobs and professions, inform themselves and other affected and interested parties of the relevant legal guidance and requirements affecting the handling and treatment of blood borne pathogens.

Athletic trainers cannot be expected to practice law or medicine, and efforts with respect to compliance with these guidelines and requirements must be commensurate with the athletic trainer's profession and professional requirements. It may be appropriate for athletic trainers to keep copies of the Center for Disease Control regulations and OSHA regulations and guidelines available for their own and others' use.

Medical Records and Confidentiality

The security, record-keeping, and confidentiality requirements and concerns that relate to athletes' medical records generally apply equally to those portions of athletes' medical records that concern blood borne pathogens.

Since social stigma is sometimes attached to individuals infected with blood borne pathogens, athletic trainers should pay particular care to the security, record-keeping, and confidentiality requirements that govern the medical records for which they have a professional obligation to see, use, keep, interpret, record, update, or otherwise handle.

Security, record-keeping, and confidentiality procedures should be maintained with respect to the records of other athletic trainers, employees, student athletic trainers, and athletes, to the extent that the athletic trainer has responsibility for these records.

The Infected Athletic Trainer

An athletic trainer infected with a blood borne pathogen should practice the profession of athletic training taking into account all professionally, medically, and legally relevant issues raised by the infection. Depending on individual circumstances, the infected athletic trainer will or may wish to:

1. Seek medical care and on-going evaluation

2. Take reasonable steps to avoid potential and identifiable risks to his or her own health and the health of his or her patients

3. Inform, as or when appropriate, relevant patients, administrators, or medical personnel

HIV and HBV Testing

Athletic trainers should follow federal, state, local and institutional laws, regulations, and guidelines concerning HIV and HBV testing. Athletic trainers should, in appropriate practice settings and situations, find it advisable to educate or assist athletes with respect to the availability of testing.

HBV Vaccinations

Consistent with professional requirements and restrictions, athletic trainers should encourage HBV vaccinations for all employees at risk, in accordance with OSHA guidelines.

Withholding of Care and Discrimination

NATA's policies and its Code of Ethics make it unethical to discriminate illegally on the basis of medical conditions.

References

1. American Academy of Pediatrics. Human immunodeficiency virus [acquired immunodeficiency syndrome (AIDS) virus] in the athletic setting. *Pediatrics.* 1991; 88:640-641.

2. American Medical Association, Department of HIV, Division of Health Science. *Digest of HIV/AIDS Policy.* Chicago, IL: Department of HIV, American Medical Association; 1993: 1-15.

3. American Medical Society for Sports Medicine and American Academy of Sports Medicine. Human immunodeficiency virus (HIV) and other blood-borne pathogens in sports. *American Journal of Sports Medicine.* In press.

4. Benson, M.T., ed. Guideline 2H: blood-borne pathogens and intercollegiate athletics. *NCAA Sports Medicine Handbook.* 1993:24-28.

5. Michigan Department of Public Health. Michigan recommendations on HBV- and/or HIV-infected health care workers. *Triad.* 1992; 4:32-34.

OSHA Guidelines on Bloodborne Pathogens

XI. The Standard

General Industry

Part 1910 of title 29 of the Code of Federal Regulations is amended as follows:

PART 1910—[AMENDED]

Subpart Z—[Amended]

1. The general authority citation for subpart Z of 29 CFR part 1910 continues to read as follows and a new citation for § 1910.1030 is added:

Authority: Secs. 6 and 8, Occupational Safety and Health Act, 29 U.S.C. 655,657, Secretary of Labor's Orders Nos. 12–71 (36 FR 8754), 8–76 (41 FR 25059), or 9–83 (48 FR 35736), as applicable; and 29 CFR part 1911.

*   *   *   *   *

Section 1910.1030 also issued under 29 U.S.C. 653.

*   *   *   *   *

2. Section 1910.1030 is added to read as follows:

§ 1910.1030   Bloodborne Pathogens.

(a) *Scope and Application.* This section applies to all occupational exposure to blood or other potentially infectious materials as defined by paragraph (b) of this section.

(b) *Definitions.* For purposes of this section, the following shall apply:

Assistant Secretary means the Assistant Secretary of Labor for Occupational Safety and Health, or designated representative.

Blood means human blood, human blood components, and products made from human blood.

Bloodborne Pathogens means pathogenic microorganisms that are present in human blood and can cause disease in humans. These pathogens include, but are not limited to, hepatitis B virus (HBV) and human immunodeficiency virus (HIV).

Clinical Laboratory means a workplace where diagnostic or other screening procedures are performed on blood or other potentially infectious materials.

Contaminated means the presence or the reasonably anticipated presence of blood or other potentially infectious materials on an item or surface.

Contaminated Laundry means laundry which has been soiled with blood or other potentially infectious materials or may contain sharps.

Contaminated Sharps means any contaminated object that can penetrate the skin including, but not limited to, needles, scalpels, broken glass, broken capillary tubes, and exposed ends of dental wires.

Decontamination means the use of physical or chemical means to remove, inactivate, or destroy bloodborne pathogens on a surface or item to the point where they are no longer capable of transmitting infectious particles and the surface or item is rendered safe for handling, use, or disposal.

Director means the Director of the National Institute for Occupational Safety and Health, U.S. Department of Health and Human Services, or designated representative.

Engineering Controls means controls (e.g., sharps disposal containers, self-sheathing needles) that isolate or remove the bloodborne pathogens hazard from the workplace.

Exposure Incident means a specific eye, mouth, other mucous membrane, non-intact skin, or parenteral contact with blood or other potentially infectious materials that results from the performance of an employee's duties.

Handwashing Facilities means a facility providing an adequate supply of running potable water, soap and single use towels or hot air drying machines.

Licensed Healthcare Professional is a person whose legally permitted scope of practice allows him or her to independently perform the activities required by paragraph (f) Hepatitis B Vaccination and Post-exposure Evaluation and Follow-up.

HBV means hepatitis B virus.

HIV means human immunodeficiency virus.

Occupational Exposure means reasonably anticipated skin, eye, mucous membrane, or parenteral contact with blood or other potentially infectious materials that may result from the performance of an employee's duties.

Other Potentially Infectious Materials means

(1) The following human body fluids: semen, vaginal secretions, cerebrospinal fluid, synovial fluid, pleural fluid, pericardial fluid, peritoneal fluid, amniotic fluid, saliva in dental procedures, any body fluid that is visibly contaminated with blood, and all body fluids in situations where it is difficult or impossible to differentiate between body fluids;

(2) Any unfixed tissue or organ (other than intact skin) from a human (living or dead); and

(3) HIV-containing cell or tissue cultures, organ cultures, and HIV- or HBV-containing culture medium or other solutions; and blood, organs, or other tissues from experimental animals infected with HIV or HBV.

Parenteral means piercing mucous membranes or the skin barrier through such events as needlesticks, human bites, cuts, and abrasions.

Personal Protective Equipment is specialized clothing or equipment worn by an employee for protection against a hazard. General work clothes (e.g., uniforms, pants, shirts or blouses) not intended to function as protection against a hazard are not considered to be personal protective equipment.

Production Facility means a facility engaged in industrial-scale, large-volume or high concentration production of HIV or HBV.

Regulated Waste means liquid or semi-liquid blood or other potentially infectious materials; contaminated items that would release blood or other potentially infectious materials in a liquid or semi-liquid state if compressed; items that are caked with dried blood or other potentially infectious materials and are capable of releasing these materials during handling; contaminated sharps; and pathological and microbiological wastes containing blood or other potentially infectious materials.

Research Laboratory means a laboratory producing or using research-laboratory-scale amounts of HIV or HBV. Research laboratories may produce high concentrations of HIV or HBV but not in the volume found in production facilities.

Source Individual means any individual, living or dead, whose blood or other potentially infectious materials may be a source of occupational exposure to the employee. Examples include, but are not limited to, hospital and clinic patients; clients in institutions for the developmentally disabled; trauma victims; clients of drug and alcohol treatment facilities; residents of hospices and nursing homes; human remains; and individuals who donate or sell blood or blood components.

Sterilize means the use of a physical or chemical procedure to destroy all microbial life including highly resistant bacterial endospores.

Universal Precautions is an approach to infection control. According to the concept of Universal Precautions, all human blood and certain human body fluids are treated as if known to be infectious for HIV, HBV, and other bloodborne pathogens.

Work Practice Controls means controls that reduce the likelihood of exposure by altering the manner in which a task is performed (e.g., prohibiting recapping of needles by a two-handed technique).

(c) *Exposure control*—(1) *Exposure Control Plan.* (i) Each employer having an employee(s) with occupational exposure as defined by paragraph (b) of this section shall establish a written Exposure Control Plan designed to eliminate or minimize employee exposure.

(ii) The Exposure Control Plan shall contain at least the following elements:

(A) The exposure determination required by paragraph (c)(2),

(B) The schedule and method of implementation for paragraphs (d) Methods of Compliance, (e) HIV and HBV Research Laboratories and Production Facilities, (f) Hepatitis B Vaccination and Post-Exposure Evaluation and Follow-up, (g) Communication of Hazards to Employees, and (h) Recordkeeping, of this standard, and

(C) The procedure for the evaluation of circumstances surrounding exposure incidents as required by paragraph (f)(3)(i) of this standard.

(iii) Each employer shall ensure that a copy of the Exposure Control Plan is accessible to employees in accordance with 29 CFR 1910.20(e).

(iv) The Exposure Control Plan shall be reviewed and updated at least annually and whenever necessary to reflect new or modified tasks and procedures which affect occupational exposure and to reflect new or revised employee positions with occupational exposure.

(v) The Exposure Control Plan shall be made available to the Assistant Secretary and the Director upon request for examination and copying.

(2) *Exposure determination.* (i) Each employer who has an employee(s) with occupational exposure as defined by paragraph (b) of this section shall prepare an exposure determination. This exposure determination shall contain the following:

(A) A list of all job classifications in which all employees in those job classifications have occupational exposure;

(B) A list of job classifications in which some employees have occupational exposure, and

(C) A list of all tasks and procedures or groups of closely related task and procedures in which occupational exposure occurs and that are performed by employees in job classifications listed in accordance with the provisions of paragraph (c)(2)(i)(B) of this standard.

(ii) This exposure determination shall be made without regard to the use of personal protective equipment.

(d) *Methods of compliance*—(1) *General*—Universal precautions shall be observed to prevent contact with blood or other potentially infectious materials. Under circumstances in which differentiation between body fluid types is difficult or impossible, all body fluids shall be considered potentially infectious materials.

(2) *Engineering and work practice controls.* (i) Engineering and work practice controls shall be used to eliminate or minimize employee exposure. Where occupational exposure remains after institution of these controls, personal protective equipment shall also be used.

(ii) Engineering controls shall be examined and maintained or replaced on a regular schedule to ensure their effectiveness.

(iii) Employers shall provide handwashing facilities which are readily accessible to employees.

(iv) When provision of handwashing facilities is not feasible, the employer shall provide either an appropriate antiseptic hand cleanser in conjunction with clean cloth/paper towels or antiseptic towelettes. When antiseptic hand cleansers or towelettes are used, hands shall be washed with soap and running water as soon as feasible.

(v) Employers shall ensure that employees wash their hands immediately or as soon as feasible after removal of gloves or other personal protective equipment.

(vi) Employers shall ensure that employees wash hands and any other skin with soap and water, or flush mucous membranes with water immediately or as soon as feasible following contact of such body areas with blood or other potentially infectious materials.

(vii) Contaminated needles and other contaminated sharps shall not be bent, recapped, or removed except as noted in paragraphs (d)(2)(vii)(A) and (d)(2)(vii)(B) below. Shearing or breaking of contaminated needles is prohibited.

(A) Contaminated needles and other contaminated sharps shall not be recapped or removed unless the employer can demonstrate that no alternative is feasible or that such action is required by a specific medical procedure.

(B) Such recapping or needle removal must be accomplished through the use of a mechanical device or a one-handed technique.

(viii) Immediately or as soon as possible after use, contaminated reusable sharps shall be placed in appropriate containers until properly reprocessed. These containers shall be:

(A) Puncture resistant;

(B) Labeled or color-coded in accordance with this standard;

(C) Leakproof on the sides and bottom; and

(D) In accordance with the requirements set forth in paragraph (d)(4)(ii)(E) for reusable sharps.

(ix) Eating, drinking, smoking, applying cosmetics or lip balm, and handling contact lenses are prohibited in work areas where there is a reasonable likelihood of occupational exposure.

(x) Food and drink shall not be kept in refrigerators, freezers, shelves, cabinets or on countertops or benchtops where blood or other potentially infectious materials are present.

(xi) All procedures involving blood or other potentially infectious materials shall be performed in such a manner as to minimize splashing, spraying, spattering, and generation of droplets of these substances.

(xii) Mouth pipetting/suctioning of blood or other potentially infectious materials is prohibited.

(xiii) Specimens of blood or other potentially infectious materials shall be placed in a container which prevents leakage during collection, handling, processing, storage, transport, or shipping.

(A) The container for storage, transport, or shipping shall be labeled or color-coded according to paragraph (g)(1)(i) and closed prior to being stored, transported, or shipped. When a facility utilizes Universal Precautions in the handling of all specimens, the labeling/color-coding of specimens is not necessary provided containers are recognizable as containing specimens. This exemption only applies while such specimens/containers remain within the facility. Labeling or color-coding in accordance with paragraph (g)(1)(i) is required when such specimens/containers leave the facility.

(B) If outside contamination of the primary container occurs, the primary container shall be placed within a second container which prevents leakage during handling, processing, storage, transport, or shipping and is labeled or color-coded according to the requirements of this standard.

(C) If the specimen could puncture the primary container, the primary container shall be placed within a secondary container which is puncture-resistant in addition to the above characteristics.

(xiv) Equipment which may become contaminated with blood or other potentially infectious materials shall be examined prior to servicing or shipping and shall be decontaminated as necessary, unless the employer can demonstrate that decontamination of such equipment or portions of such equipment is not feasible.

(A) A readily observable label in accordance with paragraph (g)(1)(i)(H) shall be attached to the equipment stating which portions remain contaminated.

(B) The employer shall ensure that this information is conveyed to all affected employees, the servicing representative, and/or the manufacturer, as appropriate, prior to handling, servicing, or shipping so that appropriate precautions will be taken.

(3) Personal protective equipment—(i) Provision. When there is occupational exposure, the employer shall provide, at no cost to the employee, appropriate personal protective equipment such as, but not limited to, gloves, gowns, laboratory coats, face shields or masks and eye protection, and mouthpieces, resuscitation bags, pocket masks, or other ventilation devices. Personal protective equipment will be considered "appropriate" only if it does not permit blood or other potentially infectious materials to pass through to or reach the employee's work clothes, street clothes, undergarments, skin, eyes, mouth, or other mucous membranes under normal conditions of use and for the duration of time which the protective equipment will be used.

(ii) Use. The employer shall ensure that the employee uses appropriate personal protective equipment unless the employer shows that the employee temporarily and briefly declined to use personal protective equipment when, under rare and extraordinary circumstances, it was the employee's professional judgment that in the specific instance its use would have prevented the delivery of health care or public safety services or would have posed an increased hazard to the safety of the worker or co-worker. When the employee makes this judgment, the circumstances shall be investigated and documented in order to determine whether changes can be instituted to prevent such occurrences in the future.

(iii) Accessibility. The employer shall ensure that appropriate personal protective equipment in the appropriate sizes is readily accessible at the worksite or is issued to employees. Hypoallergenic gloves, glove liners, powderless gloves, or other similar alternatives shall be readily accessible to those employees who are allergic to the gloves normally provided.

(iv) Cleaning, Laundering, and Disposal. The employer shall clean, launder, and dispose of personal protective equipment required by paragraphs (d) and (e) of this standard, at no cost to the employee.

(v) Repair and Replacement. The employer shall repair or replace personal protective equipment as needed to maintain its effectiveness, at no cost to the employee.

(vi) If a garment(s) is penetrated by blood or other potentially infectious materials, the garment(s) shall be removed immediately or as soon as feasible.

(vii) All personal protective equipment shall be removed prior to leaving the work area.

(viii) When personal protective equipment is removed it shall be placed in an appropriately designated area or container for storage, washing, decontamination or disposal.

(ix) Gloves. Gloves shall be worn when it can be reasonably anticipated that the employee may have hand contact with blood, other potentially infectious materials, mucous membranes, and non-intact skin; when performing vascular access procedures except as specified in paragraph (d)(3)(ix)(D); and when handling or touching contaminated items or surfaces.

(A) Disposable (single use) gloves such as surgical or examination gloves, shall be replaced as soon as practical when contaminated or as soon as feasible if they are torn, punctured, or when their ability to function as a barrier is compromised.

(B) Disposable (single use) gloves shall not be washed or decontaminated for re-use.

(C) Utility gloves may be decontaminated for re-use if the integrity of the glove is not compromised. However, they must be discarded if they are cracked, peeling, torn, punctured, or exhibit other signs of deterioration or when their ability to function as a barrier is compromised.

(D) If an employer in a volunteer blood donation center judges that routine gloving for all phlebotomies is not necessary then the employer shall:

(1) Periodically reevaluate this policy;

(2) Make gloves available to all employees who wish to use them for phlebotomy;

(3) Not discourage the use of gloves for phlebotomy; and

(4) Require that gloves be used for phlebotomy in the following circumstances:

(i) When the employee has cuts, scratches, or other breaks in his or her skin;

(ii) When the employee judges that hand contamination with blood may occur, for example, when performing phlebotomy on an uncooperative source individual; and

(iii) When the employee is receiving training in phlebotomy.

(x) Masks, Eye Protection, and Face Shields. Masks in combination with eye protection devices, such as goggles or glasses with solid side shields, or chin-length face shields, shall be worn whenever splashes, spray, spatter, or droplets of blood or other potentially infectious materials may be generated and eye, nose, or mouth contamination can be reasonably anticipated.

(xi) Gowns, Aprons, and Other Protective Body Clothing. Appropriate protective clothing such as, but not limited to, gowns, aprons, lab coats, clinic jackets, or similar outer garments shall be worn in occupational exposure situations. The type and characteristics will depend upon the task and degree of exposure anticipated.

(xii) Surgical caps or hoods and/or shoe covers or boots shall be worn in instances when gross contamination can reasonably be anticipated (e.g., autopsies, orthopaedic surgery).

(4) *Housekeeping.* (i) General. Employers shall ensure that the worksite is maintained in a clean and sanitary condition. The employer shall determine and implement an appropriate written schedule for cleaning and method of decontamination based upon the location within the facility, type of surface to be cleaned, type of soil present, and tasks or procedures being performed in the area.

(ii) All equipment and environmental and working surfaces shall be cleaned and decontaminated after contact with blood or other potentially infectious materials.

(A) Contaminated work surfaces shall be decontaminated with an appropriate disinfectant after completion of procedures; immediately or as soon as feasible when surfaces are overtly contaminated or after any spill of blood or other potentially infectious materials; and at the end of the work shift if the surface may have become contaminated since the last cleaning.

(B) Protective coverings, such as plastic wrap, aluminum foil, or imperviously-backed absorbent paper used to cover equipment and environmental surfaces, shall be removed and replaced as soon as feasible when they become overtly contaminated or at the end of the workshift if they may have become contaminated during the shift.

(C) All bins, pails, cans, and similar receptacles intended for reuse which have a reasonable likelihood for becoming contaminated with blood or other potentially infectious materials shall be inspected and decontaminated on a regularly scheduled basis and cleaned and decontaminated immediately or as soon as feasible upon visible contamination.

(D) Broken glassware which may be contaminated shall not be picked up directly with the hands. It shall be cleaned up using mechanical means, such as a brush and dust pan, tongs, or forceps.

(E) Reusable sharps that are contaminated with blood or other potentially infectious materials shall not be stored or processed in a manner that requires employees to reach by hand into the containers where these sharps have been placed.

(iii) Regulated Waste.

(A) Contaminated Sharps Discarding and Containment. (*1*) Contaminated sharps shall be discarded immediately or as soon as feasible in containers that are:

(*i*) Closable;

(*ii*) Puncture resistant;

(*iii*) Leakproof on sides and bottom; and

(*iv*) Labeled or color-coded in accordance with paragraph (g)(1)(i) of this standard.

(2) During use, containers for contaminated sharps shall be:

(*i*) Easily accessible to personnel and located as close as is feasible to the immediate area where sharps are used or can be reasonably anticipated to be found (e.g., laundries);

(*ii*) Maintained upright throughout use; and

(*iii*) Replaced routinely and not be allowed to overfill.

(3) When moving containers of contaminated sharps from the area of use, the containers shall be:

(*i*) Closed immediately prior to removal or replacement to prevent spillage or protrusion of contents during handling, storage, transport, or shipping;

(*ii*) Placed in a secondary container if leakage is possible. The second container shall be:

(*A*) Closable;

(*B*) Constructed to contain all contents and prevent leakage during handling, storage, transport, or shipping; and

(*C*) Labeled or color-coded according to paragraph (g)(1)(i) of this standard.

(*4*) Reusable containers shall not be opened, emptied, or cleaned manually or in any other manner which would expose employees to the risk of percutaneous injury.

(B) Other Regulated Waste Containment. (*1*) Regulated waste shall be placed in containers which are:

(*i*) Closable;

(*ii*) Constructed to contain all contents and prevent leakage of fluids during handling, storage, transport or shipping;

(*iii*) Labeled or color-coded in accordance with paragraph (g)(1)(i) this standard; and

(*iv*) Closed prior to removal to prevent spillage or protrusion of contents during handling, storage, transport, or shipping;

(*2*) If outside contamination of the regulated waste container occurs, it shall be placed in a second container. The second container shall be:

(*i*) Closable;

(*ii*) Constructed to contain all contents and prevent leakage of fluids during handling, storage, transport, or shipping;

(*iii*) Labeled or color-coded in accordance with paragraph (g)(1)(i) of this standard; and

(*iv*) Closed prior to removal to prevent spillage or protrusion of contents during handling, storage, transport, or shipping.

(C) Disposal of all regulated waste shall be in accordance with applicable regulations of the United States, States and Territories, and political subdivisions of States and Territories.

(iv) Laundry.

(A) Contaminated laundry shall be handled as little as possible with a minimum of agitation. (1) Contaminated laundry shall be bagged or containerized at the location where it was used and shall not be sorted or rinsed in the location of use.

(2) Contaminated laundry shall be placed and transported in bags or containers labeled or color-coded in accordance with paragraph (g)(1)(i) of this standard. When a facility utilizes Universal Precautions in the handling of all soiled laundry, alternative labeling or color-coding is sufficient if it permits all employees to recognize the containers as requiring compliance with Universal Precautions.

(3) Whenever contaminated laundry is wet and presents a reasonable likelihood of soak-through of or leakage from the bag or container, the laundry shall be placed and transported in bags or containers which prevent soak-through and/or leakage of fluids to the exterior.

(B) The employer shall ensure that employees who have contact with contaminated laundry wear protective gloves and other appropriate personal protective equipment.

(C) When a facility ships contaminated laundry off-site to a second facility which does not utilize Universal Precautions in the handling of all laundry, the facility generating the contaminated laundry must place such laundry in bags or containers which are labeled or color-coded in accordance with paragraph (g)(1)(i).

(e) *HIV and HBV Research Laboratories and Production Facilities.* (1) This paragraph applies to research laboratories and production facilities engaged in the culture, production, concentration, experimentation, and manipulation of HIV and HBV. It does not apply to clinical or diagnostic laboratories engaged solely in the analysis of blood, tissues, or organs. These requirements apply in addition to the other requirements of the standard.

(2) Research laboratories and production facilities shall meet the following criteria:

(i) Standard microbiological practices. All regulated waste shall either be incinerated or decontaminated by a method such as autoclaving known to effectively destroy bloodborne pathogens.

(ii) Special practices.

(A) Laboratory doors shall be kept closed when working involving HIV or HBV is in progress.

(B) Contaminated materials that are to be decontaminated at a site away from the work area shall be placed in a durable, leakproof, labeled or color-coded container that is closed before being removed from the work area.

(C) Access to the work area shall be limited to authorized persons. Written policies and procedures shall be established whereby only persons who have been advised of the potential biohazard, who meet any specific entry requirements, and who comply with all entry and exit procedures shall be allowed to enter the work areas and animal rooms.

(D) When other potentially infectious materials or infected animals are present in the work area or containment module, a hazard warning sign incorporating the universal biohazard symbol shall be posted on all access doors. The hazard warning sign shall comply with paragraph (g)(1)(ii) of this standard.

(E) All activities involving other potentially infectious materials shall be conducted in biological safety cabinets or other physical-containment devices within the containment module. No work with these other potentially infectious materials shall be conducted on the open bench.

(F) Laboratory coats, gowns, smocks, uniforms, or other appropriate protective clothing shall be used in the work area and animal rooms. Protective clothing shall not be worn outside of the work area and shall be decontaminated before being laundered.

(G) Special care shall be taken to avoid skin contact with other potentially infectious materials. Gloves shall be worn when handling infected animals and when making hand contact with other potentially infectious materials is unavoidable.

(H) Before disposal all waste from work areas and from animal rooms shall either be incinerated or decontaminated by a method such as autoclaving known to effectively destroy bloodborne pathogens.

(I) Vacuum lines shall be protected with liquid disinfectant traps and high-efficiency particulate air (HEPA) filters or filters of equivalent or superior efficiency and which are checked routinely and maintained or replaced as necessary.

(J) Hypodermic needles and syringes shall be used only for parenteral injection and aspiration of fluids from laboratory animals and diaphragm bottles. Only needle-locking syringes or disposable syringe-needle units (i.e., the needle is integral to the syringe) shall be used for the injection or aspiration of other potentially infectious materials. Extreme caution shall be used when handling needles and syringes. A needle shall not be bent, sheared, replaced in the sheath or guard, or removed from the syringe following use. The needle and syringe shall be promptly placed in a puncture-resistant container and autoclaved or decontaminated before reuse or disposal.

(K) All spills shall be immediately contained and cleaned up by appropriate professional staff or others properly trained and equipped to work with potentially concentrated infectious materials.

(L) A spill or accident that results in an exposure incident shall be immediately reported to the laboratory director or other responsible person.

(M) A biosafety manual shall be prepared or adopted and periodically reviewed and updated at least annually or more often if necessary. Personnel shall be advised of potential hazards, shall be required to read instructions on practices and procedures, and shall be required to follow them.

(iii) Containment equipment. (A) Certified biological safety cabinets (Class I, II, or III) or other appropriate combinations of personal protection or physical containment devices, such as special protective clothing, respirators, centrifuge safety cups, sealed centrifuge rotors, and containment caging for animals, shall be used for all activities with other potentially infectious materials that pose a threat of exposure to droplets, splashes, spills, or aerosols.

(B) Biological safety cabinets shall be certified when installed, whenever they are moved and at least annually.

(3) HIV and HBV research laboratories shall meet the following criteria:

(i) Each laboratory shall contain a facility for hand washing and an eye wash facility which is readily available within the work area.

(ii) An autoclave for decontamination of regulated waste shall be available.

(4) HIV and HBV production facilities shall meet the following criteria:

(i) The work areas shall be separated from areas that are open to unrestricted traffic flow within the building. Passage through two sets of doors shall be the basic requirement for entry into the work area from access corridors or other contiguous areas. Physical separation of the high-containment work area from access corridors or other areas or activities may also be provided by a double-doored clothes-change room (showers may be included), airlock, or other access facility that requires passing through two sets of doors before entering the work area.

(ii) The surfaces of doors, walls, floors and ceilings in the work area shall be water resistant so that they can be easily cleaned. Penetrations in these surfaces shall be sealed or capable of being sealed to facilitate decontamination.

(iii) Each work area shall contain a sink for washing hands and a readily available eye wash facility. The sink shall be foot, elbow, or automatically operated and shall be located near the exit door of the work area.

(iv) Access doors to the work area or containment module shall be self-closing.

(v) An autoclave for decontamination of regulated waste shall be available within or as near as possible to the work area.

(vi) A ducted exhaust-air ventilation system shall be provided. This system shall create directional airflow that draws air into the work area through the entry area. The exhaust air shall not be recirculated to any other area of the building, shall be discharged to the outside, and shall be dispersed away from occupied areas and air intakes. The proper direction of the airflow shall be verified (i.e., into the work area).

(5) *Training Requirements.* Additional training requirements for employees in HIV and HBV research laboratories and HIV and HBV production facilities are specified in paragraph (g)(2)(ix).

(f) *Hepatitis B vaccination and post-exposure evaluation and follow-up—(1) General.* (i) The employer shall make available the hepatitis B vaccine and vaccination series to all employees who have occupational exposure, and post-exposure evaluation and follow-up to all employees who have had an exposure incident.

(ii) The employer shall ensure that all medical evaluations and procedures including the hepatitis B vaccine and vaccination series and post-exposure evaluation and follow-up, including prophylaxis, are:

(A) Made available at no cost to the employee;

(B) Made available to the employee at a reasonable time and place;

(C) Performed by or under the supervision of a licensed physician or by or under the supervision of another licensed healthcare professional; and

(D) Provided according to recommendations of the U.S. Public Health Service current at the time these evaluations and procedures take place, except as specified by this paragraph (f).

(iii) The employer shall ensure that all laboratory tests are conducted by an accredited laboratory at no cost to the employee.

(2) *Hepatitis B Vaccination.* (i) Hepatitis B vaccination shall be made available after the employee has received the training required in paragraph (g)(2)(vii)(I) and within 10 working days of initial assignment to all employees who have occupational exposure unless the employee has previously received the complete hepatitis B vaccination series, antibody testing has revealed that the employee is immune, or the vaccine is contraindicated for medical reasons.

(ii) The employer shall not make participation in a prescreening program a prerequisite for receiving hepatitis B vaccination.

(iii) If the employee initially declines hepatitis B vaccination but at a later date while still covered under the standard decides to accept the vaccination, the employer shall make available hepatitis B vaccination at that time.

(iv) The employer shall assure that employees who decline to accept hepatitis B vaccination offered by the employer sign the statement in appendix A.

(v) If a routine booster dose(s) of hepatitis B vaccine is recommended by the U.S. Public Health Service at a future date, such booster dose(s) shall be made available in accordance with section (f)(1)(ii).

(3) *Post-exposure Evaluation and Follow-up.* Following a report of an exposure incident, the employer shall make immediately available to the exposed employee a confidential medical evaluation and follow-up, including at least the following elements:

(i) Documentation of the route(s) of exposure, and the circumstances under which the exposure incident occurred;

(ii) Identification and documentation of the source individual, unless the employer can establish that identification is infeasible or prohibited by state or local law;

(A) The source individual's blood shall be tested as soon as feasible and after consent is obtained in order to determine HBV and HIV infectivity. If consent is not obtained, the employer shall establish that legally required consent cannot be obtained. When the source individual's consent is not required by law, the source individual's blood, if available, shall be tested and the results documented.

(B) When the source individual is already known to be infected with HBV or HIV, testing for the source individual's known HBV or HIV status need not be repeated.

(C) Results of the source individual's testing shall be made available to the exposed employee, and the employee shall be informed of applicable laws and regulations concerning disclosure of the identity and infectious status of the source individual.

(iii) Collection and testing of blood for HBV and HIV serological status;

(A) The exposed employee's blood shall be collected as soon as feasible and tested after consent is obtained.

(B) If the employee consents to baseline blood collection, but does not give consent at that time for HIV serologic testing, the sample shall be preserved for at least 90 days. If, within 90 days of the exposure incident, the employee elects to have the baseline sample tested, such testing shall be done as soon as feasible.

(iv) Post-exposure prophylaxis, when medically indicated, as recommended by the U.S. Public Health Service;

(v) Counseling; and

(vi) Evaluation of reported illnesses.

(4) *Information Provided to the Healthcare Professional.* (i) The employer shall ensure that the healthcare professional responsible for the employee's Hepatitis B vaccination is provided a copy of this regulation.

(ii) The employer shall ensure that the healthcare professional evaluating an employee after an exposure incident is provided the following information:

(A) A copy of this regulation;

(B) A description of the exposed employee's duties as they relate to the exposure incident;

(C) Documentation of the route(s) of exposure and circumstances under which exposure occurred;

(D) Results of the source individual's blood testing, if available; and

(E) All medical records relevant to the appropriate treatment of the employee including vaccination status which are the employer's responsibility to maintain.

(5) *Healthcare Professional's Written Opinion.* The employer shall obtain and provide the employee with a copy of the evaluating healthcare professional's written opinion within 15 days of the completion of the evaluation.

(i) The healthcare professional's written opinion for Hepatitis B vaccination shall be limited to whether Hepatitis B vaccination is indicated for an employee, and if the employee has received such vaccination.

(ii) The healthcare professional's written opinion for post-exposure evaluation and follow-up shall be limited to the following information:

(A) That the employee has been informed of the results of the evaluation; and

(B) That the employee has been told about any medical conditions resulting from exposure to blood or other potentially infectious materials which require further evaluation or treatment.

(iii) All other findings or diagnoses shall remain confidential and shall not be included in the written report.

(6) *Medical recordkeeping.* Medical records required by this standard shall be maintained in accordance with paragraph (h)(1) of this section.

(g) *Communication of hazards to employees—* (1) *Labels and signs.* (i) Labels. (A) Warning labels shall be affixed to containers of regulated waste, refrigerators and freezers containing blood or other potentially infectious material; and other containers used to store, transport or ship blood or other potentially infectious materials, except as provided in paragraph (g)(1)(i)(E), (F) and (G).

(B) Labels required by this section shall include the following legend:

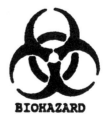

BIOHAZARD

(C) These labels shall be fluorescent orange or orange-red or predominantly so, with lettering or symbols in a contrasting color.

(D) Labels required by affixed as close as feasible to the container by string, wire, adhesive, or other method that prevents their loss or unintentional removal.

(E) Red bags or red containers may be substituted for labels.

(F) Containers of blood, blood components, or blood products that are labeled as to their contents and have been released for transfusion or other clinical use are exempted from the labeling requirements of paragraph (g).

(G) Individual containers of blood or other potentially infectious materials that are placed in a labeled container during storage, transport, shipment or disposal are exempted from the labeling requirement.

(H) Labels required for contaminated equipment shall be in accordance with this paragraph and shall also state which portions of the equipment remain contaminated.

(I) Regulated waste that has been decontaminated need not be labeled or color-coded.

(ii) Signs. (A) The employer shall post signs at the entrance to work areas specified in paragraph (e), HIV and HBV Research Laboratory and Production Facilities, which shall bear the following legend:

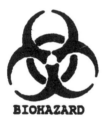

BIOHAZARD

BIOHAZARD
(Name of the Infectious Agent)
(Special requirements for entering the area)
(Name, telephone number of the laboratory director or other responsible person.)

(B) These signs shall be fluorescent orange-red or predominantly so, with lettering or symbols in a contrasting color.

(2) *Information and Training.* (i) Employers shall ensure that all employees with occupational exposure participate in a training program which must be provided at no cost to the employee and during working hours.

(ii) Training shall be provided as follows:

(A) At the time of initial assignment to tasks where occupational exposure may take place;

(B) Within 90 days after the effective date of the standard; and

(C) At least annually thereafter.

(iii) For employees who have received training on bloodborne pathogens in the year preceding the effective date of the standard, only training with respect to the provisions of the standard which were not included need be provided.

(iv) Annual training for all employees shall be provided within one year of their previous training.

(v) Employers shall provide additional training when changes such as modification of tasks or procedures or institution of new tasks or procedures affect the employee's occupational exposure. The additional training may be limited to addressing the new exposures created.

(vi) Material appropriate in content and vocabulary to educational level, literacy, and language of employees shall be used.

(vii) The training program shall contain at a minimum the following elements:

(A) An accessible copy of the regulatory text of this standard and an explanation of its contents;

(B) A general explanation of the epidemiology and symptoms of bloodborne diseases;

(C) An explanation of the modes of transmission of bloodborne pathogens;

(D) An explanation of the employer's exposure control plan and the means by which the employee can obtain a copy of the written plan;

(E) An explanation of the appropriate methods for recognizing tasks and other activities that may involve exposure to blood and other potentially infectious materials;

(F) An explanation of the use and limitations of methods that will prevent or reduce exposure including appropriate engineering controls, work practices, and personal protective equipment;

(G) Information on the types, proper use, location, removal, handling, decontamination and disposal of personal protective equipment;

(H) An explanation of the basis for selection of personal protective equipment;

(I) Information on the hepatitis B vaccine, including information on its efficacy, safety, method of administration, the benefits of being vaccinated, and that the vaccine and vaccination will be offered free of charge;

(J) Information on the appropriate actions to take and persons to contact in an emergency involving blood or other potentially infectious materials;

(K) An explanation of the procedure to follow if an exposure incident occurs, including the method of reporting the incident and the medical follow-up that will be made available;

(L) Information on the post-exposure evaluation and follow-up that the employer is required to provide for the employee following an exposure incident;

(M) An explanation of the signs and labels and/or color coding required by paragraph (g)(1); and

(N) An opportunity for interactive questions and answers with the person conducting the training session.

(viii) The person conducting the training shall be knowledgeable in the subject matter covered by the elements contained in the training program as it relates to the workplace that the training will address.

(ix) Additional Initial Training for Employees in HIV and HBV Laboratories and Production Facilities. Employees in HIV or HBV research laboratories and HIV or HBV production facilities shall receive the following initial training in addition to the above training requirements.

(A) The employer shall assure that employees demonstrate proficiency in standard microbiological practices and techniques and in the practices and operations specific to the facility before being allowed to work with HIV or HBV.

(B) The employer shall assure that employees have prior experience in the handling of human pathogens or tissue cultures before working with HIV or HBV.

(C) The employer shall provide a training program to employees who have no prior experience in handling human pathogens. Initial work activities shall not include the handling of infectious agents. A progression of work activities shall be assigned as techniques are learned and proficiency is developed. The employer shall assure that employees participate in work activities involving infectious agents only after proficiency has been demonstrated.

(h) *Recordkeeping—(1) Medical Records.* (i) The employer shall establish and maintain an accurate record for each employee with occupational exposure, in accordance with 29 CFR 1910.20.

(ii) This record shall include:

(A) The name and social security number of the employee;

(B) A copy of the employee's hepatitis B vaccination status including the dates of all the hepatitis B vaccinations and any medical records relative to the employee's ability to receive vaccination as required by paragraph (f)(2);

(C) A copy of all results of examinations, medical testing, and follow-up procedures as required by paragraph (f)(3);

(D) The employer's copy of the healthcare professional's written opinion as required by paragraph (f)(5); and

(E) A copy of the information provided to the healthcare professional as required by paragraphs (f)(4)(ii)(B)(C) and (D).

(iii) Confidentiality. The employer shall ensure that employee medical records required by paragraph (h)(1) are:

(A) Kept confidential; and

(B) Are not disclosed or reported without the employee's express written consent to any person within or outside the workplace except as required by this section or as may be required by law.

(iv) The employer shall maintain the records required by paragraph (h) for at least the duration of employment plus 30 years in accordance with 29 CFR 1910.20.

(2) *Training Records. (i) Training records shall include the following information:*

(A) The dates of the training sessions;

(B) The contents or a summary of the training sessions;

(C) The names and qualifications of persons conducting the training; and

(D) The names and job titles of all persons attending the training sessions.

(ii) Training records shall be maintained for 3 years from the date on which the training occurred.

(3) *Availability.* (i) The employer shall ensure that all records required to be maintained by this section shall be made available upon request to the Assistant Secretary and the Director for examination and copying.

(ii) Employee training records required by this paragraph shall be provided upon request for examination and copying to employees, to employee representatives, to the Director, and to the Assistant Secretary in accordance with 29 CFR 1910.20.

(iii) Employee medical records required by this paragraph shall be provided upon request for examination and copying to the subject employee, to anyone having written consent of the subject employee, to the Director, and to the Assistant Secretary in accordance with 29 CFR 1910.20.

(4) *Transfer of Records.* (i) The employer shall comply with the requirements involving transfer of records set forth in 29 CFR 1910.20(h).

(ii) If the employer ceases to do business and there is no successor employer to receive and retain the records for the prescribed period, the employer shall notify the Director, at least three months prior to their disposal and transmit them to the Director, if required by the Director to do so, within that three month period.

(i) *Dates—(1) Effective Date.* The standard shall become effective on March 6, 1992.

(2) The Exposure Control Plan required by paragraph (c)(2) of this section shall be completed on or before May 5, 1992.

(3) Paragraph (g)(2) Information and Training and (h) Recordkeeping shall take effect on or before June 4, 1992.

(4) Paragraphs (d)(2) Engineering and Work Practice Controls, (d)(3) Personal Protective Equipment, (d)(4) Housekeeping, (e) HIV and HBV Research Laboratories and Production Facilities, (f) Hepatitis B Vaccination and Post-Exposure Evaluation and Follow-up, and (g)(1) Labels and Signs, shall take effect July 6, 1992.

Appendix A to Section 1910.1030—Hepatitis B Vaccine Declination (Mandatory)

I understand that due to my occupational exposure to blood or other potentially infectious materials I may be at risk of acquiring hepatitis B virus (HBV) infection. I have been given the opportunity to be vaccinated with hepatitis B vaccine, at no charge to myself. However, I decline hepatitis B vaccination at this time. I understand that by declining this vaccine, I continue to be at risk of acquiring hepatitis B, a serious disease. If in the future I continue to have occupational exposure to blood or other potentially infectious materials and I want to be vaccinated with hepatitis B vaccine, I can receive the vaccination series at no charge to me.

[FR Doc. 91-28886 Filed 12-2-91; 8:45 am]
BILLING CODE 4510-26-M

AMSSM and AASM Joint Position Statement: HIV and Other Bloodborne Pathogens in Sports

The American Medical Society for Sports Medicine (AMSSM) and the American Academy of Sports Medicine (AASM)

The AMSSM and the AASM recognize that human immunodeficiency virus (HIV) infection and other blood-borne pathogens, including hepatitis B and C, pose a series of important and complex issues for practitioners involved in the care of athletes. This document is directed toward physicians and other health-care providers involved in the field of sports medicine and is intended to serve as a guideline to (a) understand HIV and other blood-borne pathogens as they relate to sports; (b) implement practical preventive measures that further minimize the low risk of transmission of these pathogens; (c) develop effective educational initiatives regarding these infections, their transmission, and prevention among athletes and others involved in sports; and (d) provide guidance for the care of HIV-infected athletes.

The AMSSM and AASM recognize that the medical information concerning blood-borne pathogens, particularly with regard to HIV, is evolving rapidly. This document is intended only as a guideline and is based on the present available knowledge. The following recommendations may change in the future.

HIV and Hepatitis B, C, and D: Epidemiology and Transmission

In the United States alone it is estimated that there are approximately one million HIV-infected persons. This translates into one infection in every 250 Americans.

The natural history of HIV infection, while continuously being refined, is one of a progressive disease leading to immune suppression and the development of acquired immunodeficiency syndrome (AIDS). The AIDS is characterized by the development of opportunistic infections and malignancies that ultimately lead to the death of the infected person. However, the course of the infection is frequently protracted, affording the HIV-infected person many years of good health, during which issues concerning an infected person's involvement in exercise and sports may arise.

The HIV is transmitted through sexual contact, parenteral exposure to blood and blood components, contamination of infected blood into open wounds or mucous membranes, and perinatally from an infected mother to fetus or infant. There is no evidence of transmission via other routes, such as through casual contact in a household or the aerosol route. One case was reported of transmission from an HIV-infected hemophiliac to his twin hemophiliac brother, which may have resulted from a shared razor (11). A second case was documented of transmission of the HIV from an HIV-infected child to an HIV-seronegative child. Although the mode of transmission is unknown, it is believed to be through unrecognized exposure to blood (7). Although the virus may be present in a variety of body fluids, only blood poses any degree of risk of transmission in athletic settings. Tears, sweat, urine, sputum, vomitus, saliva, and respiratory droplets have not been implicated in infection transmission.

There are currently estimated to be over one million carriers of hepatitis B virus (HBV) in the United States. Hepatitis B is spread through the same routes as HIV (sexual contact, parenteral blood exposure, and perinatally) but is more readily transmitted than HIV. Explanations for this difference may include the fact that HBV is far more concentrated in blood, with a milliliter of blood containing upward of 100 million infectious doses of the virus (4), whereas HIV is generally found in concentrations of only a few hundred to a few thousand particles per milliliter of blood (13).

In 1989, hepatitis C virus (HCV) was isolated and identified as an important cause of posttransfusion hepatitis. The current state of medical knowledge of HCV in comparison with HIV and HBV is incomplete, but it does appear to be efficiently transmitted by blood transfusion and by needle sharing among intravenous drug users, but only rarely as a result of occupational exposure in health-care settings (18).

Hepatitis delta virus (HDV) is an unusual RNA virus that requires the presence of HBV for expression of the disease. The HDV results in a more virulent course of the disease than does HBV alone and may be present during initial infection with HBV or may infect persons with preexisting HBV infection. Risk factors for the two diseases are similar (16).

Transmission of HIV and Other Blood-Borne Pathogens Through Sports

HIV

At present there are no epidemiologic studies assessing the transmission of HIV or other blood-borne pathogens during athletic activity. One alleged case of HIV transmission was reported in 1990 between soccer players in Italy (2). However, this case lacked sufficient documentation to be considered a transmission during athletic activity (3). This absence of documented cases of transmission during athletic activity is significant in view of the known prevalence of HIV infection. The risk of HIV transmission on the field in the National Football League has been conservatively estimated at below one per million games (8). The experience gathered from occupational exposure in the health-care setting has shown that the risk of transmission for parenteral exposure is likely influenced by a variety of factors, including the size of the inoculum and the route of entry. The HIV transmission is documented to occur in approximately 1 of 300 needle-stick injuries involving infected blood. However, most cases have been associated with deep (intramuscular) penetrations with hollow-bore needles (9). Mucocutlaneous transmission has been only rarely reported, and each case has involved large quantities of blood, prolonged exposure, and a portal of entry. Prospective analysis of cases of HIV-infected blood contact with mucous membranes or nonintact skin or both has shown one case of such transmission (14). These occupational data provide strong presumptive evidence that sports-related transmission of HIV is unlikely. However, despite the negative data, the theoretical chance is not zero for HIV transmission in situations in sports in which significant blood exposures to open wounds could occur. However, the risk is sufficiently small that we are not able to quantify it.

HBV

There has been one valid report (based on epidemiologic evidence) of HBV transmission in sports participation. This involved a group of high school-aged Sumo wrestlers in Japan and was reported in 1982 (15). Given the prevalence of chronic carriers of HBV in the general population, it is remarkable that only one well-validated case has been reported in the literature. In the health-care setting the risk of transmission for parenteral exposure is much greater than that of HIV (approximately three of 10) (4). In addition, cases of transmission among household/institutional contacts who have not been involved in shared needle use or sexual intercourse with other infected partners have been reported only rarely (1,12). Although not certain, the routes of entry may have resulted from unnoticed wound or mucous membrane exposure through shared razors or toothbrushes. The chronic HBV carrier who is e-antigen positive presents the greatest concern for transmission. Again, as in the case of HIV, we are not able to quantify the risk of transmission in sports. However, given the limited data about transmission, it may be presumed that the sports-related transmission risk for HBV (especially in the presence of e-antigen positive persons) is greater than the risk for HIV.

It should be recognized that contact and collision sports have a higher risk of significant blood exposure than do other sports. Athletes competing in such sports need to be aware of the small theoretical risk of blood-borne pathogen transmission in these sports. The infected athlete has special responsibilities in continuing to participate in this form of competition.

Even given these small probabilities of transmission, where preventive actions (which are consistent with basic good hygiene) are practical and simple to implement, such actions should be taken. The greatest risk to the athlete for contracting any blood-borne pathogen infection is through sexual activity and parenteral drug use, not in the sporting arena.

Education

The AMSSM and AASM recognize that preventive education remains the most important weapon in the effort to prevent blood-borne pathogen transmission. Sports medicine practitioners should play an important role in educational activities directed at athletes, their families, athletic trainers, other health-care providers, coaches, officials, and others involved in sports. First and foremost, athletes should be educated in clear and effective language about the risk of HIV and other blood-borne pathogen transmission through sexual contact. Abstinence or monogamous sex between uninfected partners is the only certain strategy for protection against sexual transmission. In other sexual relationships, the use of condoms with water-based lubricants is recommended. Although the effectiveness of spermicides containing nonoxynol-9 is still being reviewed, these may serve as adjuncts to condoms. Also, the athlete is susceptible to transmission via shared contaminated needles and syringes associated with drug use. This includes the use of ergogenic aids such as anabolic steroids as well as drugs of abuse, such as heroin. These risks should be clearly presented to the athlete as well. Athletes should also avoid sharing personal items such as razors, toothbrushes, and nail clippers.

Education regarding the risk of transmission during athletic competition is also important. The risk of such transmission, although highly improbable, can be minimized further by such common-sense hygienic measures as the prompt application of first aid to bleeding injuries. Athletes should be made aware that it is in their best interest to report significant injuries in a timely manner to the appropriate official, coach, or caregiver. Caregivers should be trained in and adhere to universal precautions (5,12).

Physicians involved in sports medicine can also play important roles in general education designed to reduce fear and misconceptions among athletes, their families, and all persons associated with sports concerning blood-borne pathogen transmission.

The athletic setting affords unique opportunities for educational initiatives regarding the transmission and prevention of HIV and other blood-borne pathogens. Physician-athlete interactions such as preparticipation or injury evaluations may be the only interactions that the athlete has with a knowledgeable health professional. Opportunities to incorporate education on disease transmission during these encounters should be sought. Athletic organizations, as well as individual athletes, may also be able to make meaningful contributions to the community's overall education effort.

The HIV-Infected Athlete

Physicians involved in sports medicine must be knowledgeable in the issues surrounding management of HIV-infected athletes. Given the continuing epidemic of HIV infection worldwide, this disease will be diagnosed in increasing numbers of infected athletes. Although HIV is an extremely serious health problem, it must be recognized that it is a chronic disease, frequently affording the infected person many years of excellent health and productive life during its natural history. During the period of preserved health, the sports medicine practitioner may be involved in the series of complex issues surrounding the advisability of continued exercise and athletic competition. The first priority of the HIV-infected athlete is ensuring that he or she comes under the care of a physician knowledgeable in the management of HIV infection. In addition, the infected athlete should be directed to appropriate counselling services dealing with the psychosocial aspects of this disease. Confidentiality of the patient must be maintained as dictated by medical ethics and legal statutes. The decision to advise continued athletic competition should be individualized involving the athlete, the athlete's personal physician, and the sports medicine practitioner. Variables to be considered in reaching this decision include (a) the athletes' current state of health and the status of the HIV infection, (b) the nature and intensity of training, (c) potential contribution of stress from athletic competition, and (d) potential risk of HIV transmission.

There is no evidence that exercise and training of moderate intensity are deleterious to the health of HIV-infected persons. To the contrary, there is growing evidence that such form of physical activity may be beneficial both psychologically and immunologically, and thus should be encouraged with appropriate monitoring (2). When counselling the HIV-infected athlete, sports medicine physicians should remember that severe psychological and physical stress, as can be found in athletic competition, can have a deleterious effect on the functions of the immune system as well as the overall state of mental and physical health and thus should be taken into consideration.

Based on current medical and epidemiologic information, HIV infection alone is insufficient grounds to prohibit athletic competition.

The HBV-Infected Athlete

In general, acute HBV infection should be viewed just as other viral infections. Decisions regarding ability to play are made according to clinical signs and symptoms such as fever, fatigue, or hepatomegaly. There is no evidence that intense, highly competitive training is a problem for the asymptomatic HBV carrier (acute or chronic).

HIV Testing

Mandatory Testing

The AMSSM and AASM believe that mandatory testing or widespread blood-borne pathogen screening is not justified for medical reasons as a condition for athletic participation or competition. Such testing would not effectively prevent infection, promote health, or be easily implemented.

Any consideration of a blood-borne pathogen testing program in the athletic setting must address the practical, medical, scientific, legal, and ethical problems that such a program poses. First, the issue of who should be tested may be unclear. Testing at one level (the professional level) cannot be done without consideration of testing at other levels (e.g., collegiate, high school, community sports programs). In addition, the frequency of testing would have to be determined. An athlete with a negative test at the beginning of the season would not be guaranteed of having a negative test 3 months later. Massive screening in low-prevalence populations leads to a higher rate of false-positive tests, resulting in undue duress, counselling, and complex follow-up evaluation. Most importantly, any testing program, no matter how widespread, is not justifiable precisely because it fails to further diminish the "too low to qualify" risk of blood-borne pathogen transmission in sports. Other factors, including overwhelming costs, as well as legal and ethical considerations of mandatory testing for populations that may include minors, further suggest that there is no rational basis for supporting blood-borne pathogen tests in sports.

Voluntary Testing

Voluntary testing should be suggested to athletes as well as nonathletes who may have been exposed to blood-borne pathogen transmission. Included would be those who have had (a) multiple sexual partners; (b) injections of nonprescription drugs, such as drugs of abuse or ergogenic aids; (c) sexual contacts with at-risk persons; (d) sexually transmitted diseases, including HBV; and (e) blood transfusions before 1985.

Pre- and posttest counselling is extremely important for anyone undergoing HIV testing and should be arranged by the ordering physician. When obtaining informed consent and reviewing the positive and negative results, state guidelines must be followed. (Guidelines may vary from state to state.)

Personal knowledge of blood-borne serum status combined with pre- and posttest counselling can be a helpful adjunct to preventive education. Knowledge of one's infection is helpful for a variety of reasons. These reasons include availability of therapy for asymptomatic patients in the case of HIV, modification of behavior that can prevent transmission of blood-borne pathogens to others, and appropriate counselling regarding exercise and sports participation. The AMSSM and AASM urge that applicable public health measures for handling an epidemic be followed with the HIV-infected persons.

Specific Management and Preventive Measures for Sports Events

Any risk of blood-borne pathogen transmission in sports is exceedingly small. However, all involved with sports will help further reduce the risk of transmission by following guidelines that are both practical and simple to implement. A major component to these guidelines is common sense and adherence to basic principles of hygiene. Universal precautions, developed by the Centers for Disease Control and Prevention, should be learned and followed by all health-care providers.

Because the risk of blood-borne pathogen transmission in sports is confined to contact with blood, body fluids, and other fluids containing blood, preventive measures should be focused on the recognition and immediate treatment of bleeding.

The following recommendations are designed to minimize the risk of blood-borne pathogen transmission in the context of athletic events and provide treatment guidelines for caregivers.

1. Preevent preparation includes proper care for existing wounds. Abrasions, cuts, or oozing wounds that may serve as a source of bleeding or as a portal of entry for blood-borne pathogens should be covered with an occlusive dressing that will withstand the demands of competition. Likewise, care providers with healing wounds or dermatitis should have these areas adequately covered to prevent transmission to or from a patient.

2. Necessary equipment or supplies or both important for compliance with universal precautions should be available to caregivers. These supplies include latex or vinyl gloves, disinfectant, bleach (freshly prepared in a 1:10 dilution with tap water), antiseptic, designated receptacles for soiled equipment or uniforms (with separate waterproof bags or receptacles appropriately marked for uniforms and equipment contaminated with blood), bandages or dressings, and a container for appropriate disposal of needles, syringes, or scalpels.

3. During the sports event, early recognition of uncontrolled bleeding is the responsibility of officials, athletes, and medical personnel. Participants with active bleeding should be removed from the event as soon as this is practical. Bleeding must be controlled and the wound cleansed with soap and water or an antiseptic. The wound must be covered with an occlusive dressing that will withstand the demands of the activity. When bleeding is controlled and any wound properly covered, the player may return to competition. Any participant whose uniform is saturated with blood, regardless of the source, must have that uniform changed before returning to competition.

4. The athletes should be advised that it is their responsibility to report all wounds and injuries in a timely manner, including those recognized before the sporting activity. It is also the athlete's responsibility to wear appropriate protective equipment at all times, including mouth protectors, in contact sports.

5. The care provider managing an acute blood exposure must follow the guidelines of universal precautions (1,15). Appropriate gloves should be worn when direct contact with blood, body fluids, and other fluids containing blood can be anticipated. Gloves should be changed after treating each individual participant and, as soon as practical after glove removal, hands should be washed with soap and water or antiseptic.

6. Minor cuts or abrasions or both commonly occur during sports. These types of wounds do not require interruption of play or removal of the participant from competition. Minor cuts and abrasions that are not bleeding should be cleansed and covered during scheduled breaks in play. Likewise, small amounts of blood stain on a uniform do not require removal of the participant or a uniform change.

7. Lack of protective equipment should not delay emergency care for life-threatening injuries. Although HIV is not transmitted by saliva, medical personnel may prefer using airway devices. These devices should be made available whenever possible.

8. Any equipment or area (e.g., wrestling mat) soiled with blood should be wiped immediately with paper towels or disposable cloths. The contaminated areas should be disinfected with a solution prepared with one part household bleach to ten parts water and should be prepared fresh daily. The cleaned area should be dry before reuse. Persons cleaning equipment or collecting soiled linen should wear gloves.

9. Postevent considerations should include re-evaluation of any wounds sustained during the sporting event. Further cleaning and dressing of the wound may be necessary. Also, blood-soiled uniforms or towels should be collected for eventual washing in hot water and detergent.

10. Procedures performed in the training room are also governed by adherence to universal precautions. Gloves should be worn by care providers. Any blood, body fluids, or other fluids containing blood should be cleaned in a manner as described previously. Equipment handlers, laundry personnel, and janitorial staff should be advised to wear gloves whenever contact with bloody equipment, clothing, or other items is anticipated. Appropriate containers for the disposal of needles, syringes, or scalpels should be available.

11. Some of the members of the athletic health-care team may be considered to be covered under OSHA guidelines. Assessment of the application of these guidelines must be made on an individual basis. This application may include consideration for HBV immunization for some personnel who are involved with the athletic health-care team. No recommendation has been specifically made for the immunizations against HBV for athletes in particular. However, several groups now recommend universal immunization against HBV of the newborn and college-aged groups (6,10,17).

Many athletic contests and practices, especially at the community or scholastic level, occur without medical personnel in attendance. The above guidelines apply not only to physicians, athletic trainers, and physical therapists involved in the coverage of sports, but also to coaches and officials who may be involved as the primary caregivers in many circumstances. All personnel involved with sports should be trained in basic first aid and infection control, including the preventive measures outlined here.

Legal Considerations

The AMSSM and AASM support the following statements regarding confidentiality and other legal considerations.

1. Confidentiality dictates that medical information is the property of the patient. The patient (or parent or guardian, in the case of a minor) is the sole decider as to whom the medical information is transmitted. Exceptions include medical conditions that are reportable by state regulation and statute. The AIDS and hepatitis A and B are reportable in all states, but HIV infections are reportable to public health agencies in many, but not all, states. Any physician who wants to know how to report a case or has related questions may contact city, county, or state health officials.

2. The team physician may feel dual, and at times conflicting, responsibilities in managing the HIV-infected athlete and other teammates or opponents. However, confidentiality makes the physician's responsibilities very clear. The physician may not apprise other physicians, coaches, trainers, teammates, or opponents of the HIV-positive athlete as to that athlete's infection. Thus, the physician is not liable for failure to warn the uninfected opponent. That legal responsibility lies with the HIV-infected athlete. However, the uninfected athlete must be aware that he or she assumes some of the risk (albeit small) of contacting HIV or other blood-borne pathogen disease in sports activities because it cannot be assumed that his or her competitors are HIV (or other blood-borne pathogen) free.

This is the same as with other injuries that are inherent in sports.

3. The courts have universally found that the responsibility for the sexual transmission of HIV lies with the HIV-infected person. As yet, there has been no legal activity regarding the transmission of HIV in athletic competition. There is then no legal precedent with regard to HIV transmission in sports.

4. The physician is advised to be aware of state and federal statutes and regulations concerning confidentiality. It is also important for the physician to know state and federal rules and regulations concerning blood contamination in the work place, including federal and state OSHA regulations on the prevention of blood-borne pathogen transmission in the work place.

References

1. *Belshe Textbook of Human Virology.* Littleton, MA: PSG Publishing, 1984:736-9.

2. Brown, L.S., Drotman, P. What is the risk of HIV infection in athletic competition? (Abstract). Presented at the 9th International Conference on AIDS, Berlin, June 6-11, 1993.

3. Calabrese, L., LaPierre, D. HIV infections: Exercise in athletes. *Sports Med* 1993;15:1-7.

4. Centers for Disease Control. Guidelines for prevention of transmission of human immunodeficiency virus and hepatitis B virus to health care and public safety workers. *MMWR* 1989;38 (suppl. 6)1-37.

5. Centers for Disease Control. Recommendations for prevention of HIV transmission in health care settings. *MMWR* 1987;36(suppl. 2) 1F-18F.

6. Committee on Infectious Diseases (American Academy of Pediatrics). Universal hepatitis B immunization. *Pediatrics* 1992;B9:795-800.

7. Fitzgibbon, J.E., Gaur, S., Frenkel, L.D., et al. Transmission from one child to another of human immunodeficiency virus type I with a zidovudine-resistance mutation. *N Engl J Med* 1993;329:1835-41.

8. Goldsmith, M. When sports and HIV share the bill. Smart money goes on common sense. *JAMA* 1992;267:1311-4.

9. Henderson, D.K., Fahey, B., Wily, M., et al. Risk for occupational transmission of human immunodeficiency virus type I (HIV-1) associated with clinical exposures. *Ann Intern Med* 1990;113:740-6.

10. Hepatitis B virus: A comprehensive strategy for eliminating transmission in the United States through universal childhood vaccination. Recommendations of the Immunization Practices Advisory Committee (ACIP). *MMWR* 1991;40:1-25.

11. HIV transmission between two adolescent brothers with hemophilia. *MMWR* 1993;42:948-51.

12. Ho, D., Moudgill, T., Alam, M. Universal precautions for prevention of transmission of human immunodeficiency virus, hepatitis B virus and other blood borne pathogens in health care settings. *MMWR* 1988;37:377-82, 387-8.

13. Ho, D., Moudgill, T., Alam, M. Quantitation of human immunodeficiency virus type I in the blood of infected persons. *N Engl J Med* 1989; 321:1621-5.

14. Ippolito, G., Puro, V., DeCarli, G., and the Italian Study Group on Occupational Risk of HIV Infection. The risk of occupational human immunodeficiency virus infection in health care workers. *Arch Intern Med* 1993;153:1451-4.

15. Kashiwagi, S. Outbreak of hepatitis B in members of a high school wrestling club. *JAMA* 1982;248:213-4.

16. Rizecio, M. The delta agent. *Hepatology* 1983;3:729-37.

17. Task Force on Vaccine Preventable Disease (American College Health Association), Institutional statement on hepatitis B vaccination. Baltimore, MD, 1993.

18. Wormser, G., Forseter, G., Joline C., et al. Hepatitis C infection in the health care setting. 1. Low risk from parenteral exposure to blood of human immunodeficiency virus-affectations. *Am J Infect Control* 1991;19:237-42.

Suggested Readings

American Academy of Pediatrics Committee on Sports Medicine Fitness. Human immunodeficiency virus (acquired immunodeficiency syndrome (AIDS)) in the athletic setting. *Pediatrics* 1991;88:640-1.

The Canadian Academy of Sports Medicine Position Statement. HIV as it relates to sport. *Clin J Sport Med* 1993;3:63-8.

NCAA Committee on Competitive Safeguards and Medical Aspects of Sports. Blood borne pathogens and intercollegiate athletics. In: *NCAA Sports Medicine Handbook.* Overland Park, KS: NCAA, 1993.

World Health Organization, International Federation of Sports Medicine. Consensus statement on AIDS in sports. Created at the World Health Organization's Global Program for AIDS, Geneva, Switzerland, January 16, 1989.

F

CDC National AIDS Clearinghouse: Locating Information About HIV/AIDS and Sports

Considerable attention has focused on the topic of HIV/AIDS and sports ever since professional basketball star Magic Johnson's announcement of his HIV infection in November 1991. Subsequent announcements about former tennis player Arthur Ashe and from Olympic diver Greg Louganis, along with news about lesser-known athletes such as former major league baseball player Glenn Burke, former hockey player Bill Goldsworthy, and boxer Lamar Parks have kept HIV/AIDS and sports in the news. While this has led to increased focus on the need for educating professional and amateur athletes, it has unfortunately also led to increased fear about the nearly nonexistent risk of transmission on the playing field.

This resource guide is intended to clear up some of the misunderstandings about HIV/AIDS and sports, and help high school, collegiate, and professional athletic personnel make informed decisions about issues related to athletics and HIV. It guides coaches, medical staff and advisors, governing boards, administrators and officials, and trainers to key resources related to HIV/AIDS and sports by listing some of the relevant issues, as well as sources for more information and assistance.

References listed following the text are footnoted throughout. Referenced articles are available through many local school, university, and public libraries. Librarians will be able to offer assistance in locating them. Policy statements, pamphlets, brochures, and other materials are available from the publishers or specified organizations. A number of these materials are available directly from the CDC National AIDS Clearinghouse (see page 90). Selected sports or health organizations listed at the back of this resource guide can provide additional assistance. A list of articles and books about professional celebrity athletes is included for those who are interested in the topic.

For those interested in locating additional information on the topic, a public library is one of the most useful tools. Within the library, the reference librarian is most often your key resource. He/she can help you locate the most useful materials for your information needs. Most communities have access to a public library; also, large research and university libraries often permit some public access to their collections. If a material that interests you is not in your library's collection, the librarian may be able to borrow it through a lending system called Interlibrary Loan.

HIV and AIDS: An Introduction

AIDS stands for acquired immunodeficiency syndrome, a disease in which the body's immune system breaks down. It is caused by human immunodeficiency virus, or HIV. Normally, the immune system protects the body against infection and other diseases. When HIV causes the immune system to fail, a person can develop a variety of life-threatening illnesses. HIV infection is a progressive disorder, often starting with a period of years during which the infected person shows no symptoms. The disease progresses slowly, sometimes taking 10 years or longer to develop into AIDS. Because of the lack of outward symptoms, HIV infection often goes undetected for months, or even years. Blood tests may detect HIV antibodies within a few weeks of the time that person becomes infected, but the "window period" between infection and the body's production of HIV antibodies can extend to six months or even a year.

About half of the people with HIV develop AIDS within 10 years, but the time between infection with HIV and the onset of AIDS can vary greatly. The severity of the HIV-related illness or illnesses differs from person to person. No cure currently exists for HIV infection or AIDS, but medical treatments can prevent, postpone, or treat many illnesses associated with AIDS. People who seek medical care to monitor and treat their HIV infection typically can carry on with their normal lifestyles, including exercising and participating in sports, for years.

HIV spreads through sexual contact with an infected person, through sharing needles with someone who is infected, or, less commonly, and now very rarely in countries where all blood donations are screened for HIV antibodies, through transfusions of infected blood or blood clotting factors. Babies born to HIV-infected women may become infected before or during birth, or through breast feeding after birth[1]. HIV is not transmitted through casual contact such as touching or sharing sports equipment and facilities.

Although HIV spreads through vaginal, anal, or oral intercourse, latex condoms prevent infection with HIV and other sexually transmitted diseases when used consistently and correctly[2]. An individual can transmit the virus to others even if he or she has no symptoms; therefore, it is important to always take precautions when having sex or sharing needles. More information about HIV and its transmission is available from the organizations listed in the back of this resource guide, or by calling the CDC National AIDS Clearinghouse at (800)458-5231.

HIV and Sports-Related Injuries

Although there is a theoretical risk of HIV transmission from an HIV-infected player to an uninfected player during athletic practice or competition[3,4], most experts agree that the risk of sports-related HIV transmission is infinitesimal[5,6,7]. Studies released by the Centers for Disease Control and Prevention (CDC) in February 1995 emphasize that the potential risk of infection during competition is extremely low, and that the principal risks faced by athletes are related to off-the-field activities[8,9]. As of March 1995, there has never been a confirmed case of HIV transmission during athletic activities. The World Health Organization (WHO), in a consensus statement developed during a consultation on AIDS and sports in Geneva on January 16, 1989, stated:

> No evidence exists for a risk of transmission of [HIV] when infected persons engaging in sports have no bleeding wounds or other skin lesions. There is no documented instances of HIV infection acquired through participation in sports. However, there is a possible very low risk of HIV transmission when one athlete who is infected has a bleeding wound or a skin lesion with exudate and another athlete has a skin lesion or exposed mucous membrane that could possibly serve as a portal of entry for the virus[10].

A soccer player in Italy reportedly contracted HIV after a bloody collision with an HIV-infected player in 1989[11]. However, the actual method of transmission remains undetermined, and experts agree that this case is not conclusive because other routes of transmission were not excluded and athletic activity could not be established as the source of infection[5,12].

HIV is not transmitted through casual contact such as touching, rubbing, sharing sports equipment or utensils, or using the same locker room or bathroom facilities. HIV is not transmitted through sweat[13] or saliva; the virus has never been identified in sweat and has been found only rarely and in minute concentrations in saliva. HIV is not transmitted by mosquitoes or other insects, through swimming pool water, or through the air[1,10,14].

HIV Transmission and Steroid Use

Sharing needles or syringes with an HIV-infected person even once presents a significant risk of becoming infected with HIV. The virus from an infected person can remain in a needle or syringe and then be injected directly into the next person who uses the needle. Injectable drugs include steroids, hormones, and vitamins.

Experts agree that there is a risk of HIV infection from sharing needles used to inject steroids[5,15,17], and that steroid use among adolescents is rising[16,17]. Two cases have been reported in which bodybuilders who shared needles to inject steroids became infected with HIV[18]. Detailed personal histories revealed that neither individual had participated in any other risk behaviors. Injectable human growth hormone, a naturally occurring hormone that is hard to detect, is becoming a popular substitute for banned steroids[14] despite the dangers of using it for such a purpose. Sharing needles to inject hormones presents the same risk for transmission of HIV. All injections should be given under medical supervision with never-used, sterile, disposable equipment.

For those who continue to inject any drug or other substance outside medical supervision, the Centers for Disease Control and Prevention (CDC), the Center for Substance Abuse Treatment, and the National Institute on Drug Abuse have issued provisional guidelines for cleaning needles[19,20]; the guidelines are available from the CDC National AIDS Clearinghouse (see page 90).

Substance Abuse and the Student-Athlete

A national study on the substance use and abuse habits of college student-athletes conducted in September 1993 showed that respondents were well-informed about the risks of HIV transmission, but that they still engaged in risky behaviors[21].

HIV-Infected Players and Participation in Sports

HIV-infected individuals can participate in sports. In fact, exercise is encouraged for many HIV-infected individuals. Each HIV-infected athlete's case should be judged on an individual basis depending on the overall physical and mental health of the player and the nature of the sport he or she plays; the athlete, doctor, trainer, and coach should make this decision together[5,22].

HIV Policy for Athletic Organizations

Based on the evidence that HIV is unlikely to be transmitted during athletics, experts agree that HIV-infected players should not routinely be excluded from practice or competition[5,15,22]. Athletic organizations and other organizations sponsoring sports programs should develop HIV/AIDS policies for their teams, schools, or organizations. Fortunately, considerable work has already been done, so no organization need start from scratch. WHO, the American Academy of Pediatrics, the National Collegiate Athletic Association (NCAA), and the Target Federation have all published scientifically sound policy statements[10,15,22,23,24]. Establishing policies regarding HIV status, participation, testing, and the handling of blood allows policymakers to make impartial, objective decisions before being confronted directly by such issues. All team and staff members should be informed of the policies so they know the guidelines under which they are working.

Precautions for Handling Blood

The theoretical risk of HIV transmission through sports activity is minute. Still, anyone coming into contact with blood from a sports-related injury should follow universal precautions. These precautions for handling blood are spelled out in the Occupational Safety and Health Administration (OSHA) regulations[25], the WHO Consensus Statement[10], the *NCAA Sports Medicine Handbook*[24], and the CDC guidelines[20,26,27]. Sports medicine personnel should familiarize themselves with this information.

HIV Testing of Players

The issue of mandatory HIV testing of athletes has arisen in discussions of HIV and sports. Most professional and collegiate athletic organizations encourage, but do not require, testing. The exceptions are in boxing: HIV tests are mandatory for boxers who fight in Nevada and in the United Kingdom. The International Boxing Federation voted in 1993 to require fighters to present evidence they are not HIV-infected before title bouts[28]. Following Greg Louganis' disclosure that he was HIV-positive while competing in the 1988 Olympics, international Olympic officials said they did not expect to make any changes in their guidelines as a result. They have adopted strict procedures for dealing with open wounds, but do not mandate HIV-antibody testing for athletes[29].

According to WHO, "There is no medical or public health justification for testing or screening for HIV infection prior to participation in sports activities"[10]. Routine HIV testing of all athletes is unnecessary, impractical, unmanageable, and costly for many reasons.

However, in spite of the evidence, nearly two-thirds of college athletes participating in contact sports would support a ban restricting HIV-infected players from competition, according to the above-mentioned survey at the University of Michigan[21]. Of those athletes competing in noncontact sports, more than half agreed that players with HIV should be barred.

Athletes and AIDS: Education Programs

The primary risks to athletes of contracting HIV infection are the same as those faced by non-athletes; that is, from having unprotected sex and from sharing needles. One study found that athletes are more likely to engage in risky lifestyle behavior patterns than nonathletes[30]. Also, the physical prowess of many athletes leads them to believe that they are invincible, and so they do not take the necessary precautions to minimize risks. Some athletes put themselves further at risk by sharing needles for injecting steroids, hormones, vitamins, or illegal drugs.

All athletic organizations should educate their staff members and athletes about HIV and AIDS. Because the team physician or trainer may be the only medical professional with whom an athlete has contact, sports medical professionals have an obligation to be informed about HIV/AIDS and to educate their athletes[14].

Footnotes

[1]*Facts About the Human Immunodeficiency Virus and Its Transmission,* Centers for Disease Control and Prevention, CDC HIV/AIDS Prevention, February 1993. Available from the CDC National AIDS Clearinghouse, PO Box 6003, Rockville, MD 20849-6003, (800) 458-5231 (inventory number D318).

[2] "Update: Barrier Protection Against HIV Infection and Other Sexually Transmitted Diseases," Centers for Disease Control and Prevention, *Morbidity and Mortality Weekly Report*, August 6, 1993; 42(30):579. Available from the CDC National AIDS Clearinghouse, PO Box 6003, Rockville, MD 20849-6003, (800) 458-5231 (inventory number D445).

[3] "An Outbreak of Herpes Gladiatorum at a High School Wrestling Camp," Belongia EA, Goodman JL, Holland EJ, et al., *New England Journal of Medicine* 1991;325(13):906.

[4] "Herpes Gladiatorum" (Letter), DeBernardo R, *New England Journal of Medicine* 1991; 326(9):647.

[5] "AIDS: Assessing the Risk Among Athletes," Hamel R, *The Physician and Sportsmedicine* 1992;146(8):1437.

[6] "AIDS Becomes a Sports Issue," Gray C, *Canadian Medical Association Journal* 1992; 146(8):1437.

[7] "HIV and Sports: What Is the Risk?" Brown LS and Drotman P, IXth International Conference on AIDS, Berlin, June 1993.

[8] "Bleeding Injuries in Professional Football: Estimating the Risk for HIV Transmission," Brown LS, Drotman DP, Chu A, et al. *Annals of Internal Medicine*, February 15, 1995;122(4):271.

[9] "Transmission of Blood-Borne Pathogens during Sports: Risk and Prevention," Mast EE, Goodman RA, Bond WW, et al. *Annal of Internal Medicine*, February 15, 1995;122(4):283.

[10] *Consensus Statement From Consultation on AIDS and Sports*, World Health Organization in collaboration with International Federation of Sports Medicine, January 16, 1989 (WHO/GPA/INF/89.2). Available from the World Health Organization Global Programme on AIDS, 20 Avenue Appia, Geneva 27, CH-1211, Switzerland.

[11] "Transmission of HIV-1 Infection Via Sports Injury" (Letter), Torre D, Sampietro C, Ferraro G, et al., *The Lancet* 1990, Vol. 335, No. 8697; 335(8697): 1105.

[12] "HIV Disease and Sport" (Letters), Loveday C, Hoffman PN and Cookson BD, Quinn N, and Torre D, *The Lancet* 1990;335(8704):1532.

[13] "Absence of Infectious Human Immunodeficiency Virus Type 1 in 'Natural' Eccrine Sweat," Wormser GP, Bittker S, Forester G, et al., *Journal of Infectious Disease* 1992;165(1):155.

[14] "Educating Athletes on HIV Disease and AIDS: The Team Physician's Role," Seltzer DG, *The Physician and Sportsmedicine* 1993; 21(1):109.

[15] "Human Immunodeficiency Virus [Acquired Immunodeficiency Syndrome (AIDS) Virus] in the

Athletic Setting," American Academy of Pediatrics Committee on Sports Medicine and Fitness, *Pediatrics* 1991;88(3):640.

[16] "AIDS Knowledge in Adolescent Anabolic Steroid Users," Jones CS, Perko M, Nagy S, et al., *Journal of Health Education* 1994;25(1):19.

[17] "Multiple HIV-Risk Behaviors Among Injection-Steroid Users," Lenaway DD, Guilfoile A, and Rebchook G, *AIDS & Public Policy Journal* 1992; 7(3):184.

[18] "HIV Infection Associated With Injections of Anabolic Steroids," (Letter), Scott MJ and Scott MJ Jr., *Journal of the American Medical Association* 1989;262(2):207.

[19] *HIV/AIDS Prevention Bulletin* (Disinfection With Bleach), Centers for Disease Control and Prevention, Center for Substance Abuse Treatment, and National Institute on Drug Abuse, April 19, 1993. Available from the CDC National AIDS Clearinghouse, PO Box 6003, Rockville, MD 20849-6003, (800) 458-5231 (inventory number D292).

[20] "Notice to Readers: Use of Bleach for Disinfection of Drug Injection Equipment," Centers for Disease Control and Prevention, *Morbidity and Mortality Weekly Report* June 4, 1993;42(21). Available from Government Printing Office, Superintendent of Documents, Washington, DC 20402-9371, (202) 783-3238, or U.S. Department of Commerce, National Technical Information Service, 5285 Port Royal Road, Springfield, VA 22151, (703) 487-4650.

[21] *Second Replication of a National Study of the Substance Use and Abuse Habits of College Student-Athletes: Final Report*, September 1993, Michigan State University, Office of Medical Education Research & Development, A-209 East Fee Hall, East Lansing, MI 48824-1316, (517) 353-9656.

[22] *AIDS/Athletics: Is There a Risk?*, National Federation Target Program, Inc., 1992. Available from National Federation of State High School Associations, PO Box 20626, Kansas City, MO 64195-0626, (816) 464-5400.

[23] "Sports Rule Committees Adopt Plans for Dealing With Bleeding Athletes," 1993, Available from the National Federation of High School Associations' TARGET Program, PO Box 20626, Kansas City, MO 64195-0626, (816) 464-5400.

[24] *1995 NCAA Sports Medicine Handbook*, National Collegiate Athletic Association, Benson MT, ed. Available from the National Collegiate Athletic Association, 6201 College Blvd., Overland Park, KS 66211-2422, (913) 339-1906.

[25] *Bloodborne Pathogens Final Standard: Summary of Key Provisions*, U.S. Department of Labor, Occupational Safety and Health Administration,

Program Highlight, Fact Sheet No. OSHA 92-46, March 6, 1992. Available from the U.S. Department of Labor, Occupational Safety and Health Administration, 200 Constitution Avenue NW, Washington, DC 20210, (202) 523-9667.

[26] "Update: Universal Precautions for Prevention of Transmission of Human Immunodeficiency Virus, Hepatitis B Virus, and Other Bloodborne Pathogens in Health-Care Settings," Centers for Disease Control, *Morbidity and Mortality Weekly Report* June 4, 1988;37(24):377. Available from the CDC National AIDS Clearinghouse (inventory number D031).

[27] "Guidelines for Prevention of Transmission of Human Immunodeficiency Virus and Hepatitis B Virus to Health-Care and Public-Safety Workers," Centers for Disease Control and Prevention, *Morbidity and Mortality Weekly Report*, 1989; 38(S-6). Available from the CDC National AIDS Clearinghouse, PO Box 6003, Rockville, MD 20849-6003, (800) 458-5231. (inventory number D423).

[28] "The HIV Issues in Six Sports," sidebar to "In NBA, AIDS Appears to Faze Few," Brubaker B, Washington Post, June 13, 1993.

[29] "Doctor Says He Treated Louganis Without Gloves Because of Time," Washington Post, February 24, 1995.

[30] "Lifestyles and Health Risks of Collegiate Athletes," Nattiv A and Puffer JC, *Journal of Family Practice* 1991;33(6):585.

Resource Materials on HIV and Professional Athletes

Articles

"Magic Johnson Ends His Career, Saying He Has the AIDS Virus," New York Times, Nov. 8, 1991

"Controversies Cause Johnson to Quit Again," New York Times, Nov. 3, 1992

"AIDS Deaths Tear at Figure-Skating World" New York Times, Nov. 17, 1992

"Arthur Ashe Announces He Has AIDS; Tennis Great's Transfusion After '83 Surgery Blamed," Washington Post, April 9, 1993

"Athlete May Be Deported for Falsifying HIV Status," Washington Post, June 22, 1994

"Fanfare: Soccer," Washington Post, Dec. 12, 1994

"A Man Once Called 'King Kong' Is Now in the Grip of Disease," Philadelphia Inquirer, Jan. 17, 1995

"Cold Reality," St. Louis-Post Dispatch, Jan. 23, 1995

"Former N.H.L. Player Reveals He Has AIDS," New York Times, Feb. 13, 1995

"Louganis, Olympic Champion, Says He Has AIDS," New York Times, Feb. 23, 1995

"Breaking the Silence," (book excerpt), *People*, March 6, 1995

"Heart of the Diver," *Time*, March 6, 1995

Books

My Life, Earvin "Magic" Johnson with William Novak, 1992. Random House, 201 E. 50th St., New York, NY 10022. (212) 751-2600.

Breaking the Surface, Greg Louganis and Eric Marcus, 1995. Random House, 201 E. 50th St., New York, NY 10022. (212) 751-2600.

Organizations for Information and Assistance

American Academy of Pediatrics
141 NW. Point Boulevard
P.O. Box 927
Elk Grove Village, IL 60009
(708) 228-5005

American Alliance for Health, Physical Education, Recreation and Dance
1900 Association Drive
Reston, VA 22091
(703) 476-3400

American Sport Education Program National Center
Human Kinetics Publishers
P.O. Box 5076
Champaign, IL 61820
(217) 351-5076

American College Health Association
P.O. Box 28937
Baltimore, MD 21240-8937
(410) 859-1500

American Medical Society for Sports Medicine
7611 Elmwood Avenue, Suite 203
Middleton, WI 53562
(608) 831-4484

American Orthopaedic Society for Sports Medicine
6300 North River Road
Suite 200
Rosemont, IL 60018
(708) 292-4900

American Red Cross
HIV/AIDS Education Office
8111 Gatehouse Road
Falls Church, VA 22042
(800) 375-2040

Canadian Council of Sport Medicine
1600 James Naismith Drive, Suite 502
Gloucester, Ontario K1B 5N4
Canada
(613) 748-5671

National Collegiate Athletic Association
6201 College Boulevard
Overland Park, KS 66211-2422
(913) 339-1906

National Federation of State High School Associations
TARGET Program
P.O. Box 20626
Kansas City, MO 64195-0626
1-800-366-6667
(816) 464-5400

President's Council on Physical Fitness and Sports
701 Pennsylvania Avenue NW, Suite 250
Washington, DC 20004
(202) 272-3421

United States Olympic Committee
One Olympic Plaza
Colorado Springs, CO 80909
(719) 632-5551

World Health Organization
Global Programme on AIDS
20 Avenue Appia
1211 Geneva 27
Switzerland
011-41-22-791-2111

For more information, contact . . .

CDC National AIDS Clearinghouse
800-458-5231, 9 am-7 pm, eastern time
800-243-7012, deaf access/TDD

The Clearinghouse provides timely, accurate, and relevant information to health and other professionals working with HIV/AIDS-related issues. The Clearinghouse provides specialized HIV/AIDS information about prevention and education materials, programs, and organizations.

CDC National AIDS Hotline
English service 1-800-342-AIDS
Spanish service 1-800-344-7432
Deaf access/TDD 1-800-243-7889

The Hotline provides current and accurate information about HIV infection and AIDS to the general public 24 hours a day, 7 days a week, 365 days a year. All information is confidential.